Animal Homeopathy

Disclaimer.
This book is a result of a long time of collecting bits of information on treating
animals with homeopathic remedies. Some of the information recorded has simply
been passed on by word of mouth. The sources of some of the material here are not
even known. This book is not a scientific leader in the field, but a "flying by the seat
of the pants" guide to helping animals with homeopathy. No harm can be done by
following these guidelines, but a great deal of good can be done.
Edition 2, when it comes out, will probably be full of colour photographs, and
have its own Materia Medica. One always hopes that a benefactor will suddenly
appear, and finance the author, as it takes astonishing amounts of time and effort to
produce these text books.
The irony of this subject is that, in orthodox medicine, many medicines are tested
extensively on animals, and then used for human beings. Animal Homeopathy
remedies are tested extensively on human beings and then used on animals.

To order additional copies, please contact us.
BookSurge, LLC
www.booksurge.com
1-866-308-6235
orders@booksurge.com

Animal Homeopathy

Comprising A Homeopathic First
Response And Guide.

CJR JUTA

2005

Animal Homeopathy

Note.

Homeopathy is not a replacement for conventional veterinary practice, but a way of maintaining optimal good health, and healing many problems permanently. Homeopathy works via the emotional system, the thinking and computing mind, the instincts, the inner organs, the bones, the lungs, the muscles, sheaths, tendons and ligaments, the blood and the skin, hair, fur and feathers. In short it is a complementary adjunct to other systems and can comfortably be used in conjunction with them.

A Salient Thought.

Looking back over the years, it is amazing how many people, and how many animals and birds could have been healed, had I then known more about healing, and especially Homeopathy. Hopefully this book will assist many people in their care of other creatures. As someone wisely said, "We grow too soon old, and too late smart". So study this book now, use it as a stepping stone on your healing journey, and do not waste your years.

The History of this Book.

"Animal Homeopathy" started out free, for animal owners everywhere. It was envisaged for people with animals on their farms, domestic and wild. It was also for those with pets, whether they are guinea-pigs, budgies, pot-bellied pigs, dogs, cats, horses, camels, lamas, spouses or anything else. It was slightly extended to help in zoos, surgeries, rescue centres, rehabilitation centres and first aid posts. The concept grew to incorporate humans to some extent. (The author has a Homeopathy/Psychology/ Qigong practice).

Any animal has free attention and remedies from me, and the book is not commercial. It is designed to ease the sufferings of animals. In this lies a small paradox. Since animals cannot speak at length about themselves, animal homeopathy is frequently reduced to treating only symptoms. This is in line with orthodox medicine, where various medicines become permanently needed, thereby making fortunes for their manufacturers, possibly even killing the patients in the long run.

The true homeopath seeks the cure by snuffling out all the symptoms, not only the presenting one, and administering a remedy to cover the complete picture. When the complete picture is not available, or in emergencies, the presenting (main) symptom is treated in isolation, to ease suffering and preserve life.

All life forms have electro-magnetic fields around

them (auras), and a series of smaller ones within them ("chakras"). Sensitive healers sense when a field is not functioning properly, and heal it using various methods from homeopathy, acupuncture, massage and crystals, to name but a few.

A system can be said to be "at ease" when all is functioning well, but in a situation of "dis-ease" when all is not well. A system in the latter state cannot recognise various invaders (you can easily have a million different types of germs, viruses and bacteria, and other things attacking your body at any time), and when it does not recognise and destroy invaders, sickness and perhaps death can result. A homeopath restores the system to a state of ease, so that it recognises and destroys them. Good health, energy and happiness can be the result. Sometimes this is described as "building up the immune system".

There is, of course, a place for orthodox medicine, especially in surgery and saving of lives in emergencies, but a perspective should be maintained between the various complementary systems and orthodox approaches.

When asked to explain which animals this book applies to, and what disorders, the answer is that it enables the owner to tackle matters as diverse as bloat in a hippopotamus, airsickness in a hawk, timidity in a vulture, eczema on a rat, diarrhoea in a chicken and stress in a parrot.

Hopefully you will have many years of enjoyment and use from this book.

The Calling of the Homeopath.

My calling as a practitioner of the art of homeopathic medicine, is to encourage the Vital Force within all entities, to function as it was designed to do, so as to recognise and destroy all morbid influences which threaten its integrity and lead to disease. I undertake to respect and honour this spirit, wherever it is found, and to help restore the connection between all entities on this planet. I undertake not to accept the limitations posed by words, cultures and species, and to make my mind receptive to the greater powers and energies everywhere.

To this end I will study continuously, co-operating with the Tao, or natural flow of powers, healing each entity with individualized attention and remedies, and teaching these principles to whoever is able to understand them.

C.J.Rupert Juta 2005

People Who Should Have This Book.

Pet owners
Game farmers
Smallholders
Hikers
Campers
Climbers
Horse owners
Farmers
Cattle ranchers
Animal rehabilitation workers
Animal hospital staff
Rescue centre staff
Animal lovers
Tourists
Police
Veterinary surgeons
Circus workers
Zoo staff
Show jumpers
Race-horse owners
Ambulance drivers and nurses
Ministers of religion
Municipal office staff
Pet shop owners
Animal trainers
Animal transporters

Airport animal staff
Stockowners
Park wardens
Healers
Complementary therapists
Animal breeders
Everyone dealing with any animals
Anyone who might conceivably come into contact with distressed animals.

Patients that may benefit from Homeopathy.

Homeopathy can be of use to all mammals and birds, including human beings, aquatic creatures, and may be of use for some reptiles. Plants have been reported to respond very positively to homeopathic remedies, but the author has little knowledge of homeopathy with plants and reptiles.

Curriculum vitae 2005.

❧

Coenraad Jacobus Rupert Juta.
Born South African (Swedish/Scottish), naturalised British.

❧

Occupation History.
1. Own **Homeopathy** practice, including exercise, chi kung, psychology (active).
2. Shareholder (22yrs), very successful **game/tourist farm development**(active).
3. Hands-on **construction** business and **estate agency**, up to 120 staff, own design and construction, speculation luxury houses, earthmoving, landscaping. Contracted to Courtaulds (mainly laboratories), some private contracting and ongoing insurance claims to banks and building societies. **Disaster standby** for insurance companies. (17 years) Numerous **projects managed**. Hotel refurbishment and **Retirement Villages** (active).
4. Private Finance, **Business Plans**, analysis, marketing, corporate venturing, business angels (1980 to present).
5. **Arbitrator**, banks/law firms/building societies/ construction contracts (7yrs).
6. Water pump **manufacture**, repair, parts, **export** (part-time 8 years, still active). Also actively imported clothing, tyres and other commodities.
7. Head of Industrial, Agricultural and Commercial **training** in Kwa-Zulu Development Corporation, before government centralized control.

8. English teaching ESL, high school, 5 years, adults in construction 17 years.

9. Part-time hobby **invigilation** and marking of English

exam papers, since 1970's, culminating in being Senior Invigilator and Examiner for Cambridge University examinations at Bell Centre, still active.

Achievements.

Rotary 20 years, Gold Medal for New Club Development.

Town Counsellor, 12 years, Chief of Works, Deputy Chairman.

Military service, Commando Reaction Force 8 years.

Civil Defence part-time Fire Chief 13 years.

Flood Relief and Disaster headed crews 17 years.

Rowing captain 6 man raft, unbeaten in class 7 years.

Martial Arts, Keeper of the styles Tao-Shukokairyu and Viper Kara-Te, Black Belt Hall of Fame. **Author** of textbooks. Constantly developing styles.

M.O.T.H. (Memorable Order of Tin Hats).

Author animal homeopathy textbook and field guide.

Interests.

1.Animal welfare, comfort, protection, health.

2.Healing people in all respects, complementary therapies and psychology.

3.Dream occupation: Development of another game farm, tourism, hikes etc.

4.Comparative religions, philosophies, study, meditation, self-hypnosis.

5.Genealogy, working on own family for many decades.

6.Archaeology, Khoi and aviation archaeology (sunken airoplanes).

7.Renovation, design, sale and construction of houses, flats, hotels, retirement complexes, no highrise.

8.Counter-insurgency, security, private security, safety procedures.

Index of Diseases.

A.
Abortion.
Abdomenal distention.
Abscess.
Afterbirth.
Ageing.
Aggression.
Allergy.
Anaemia.
Anaesthesia recovery.
Anger.
Anthrax.
Anxiety.
Apathy.
Arthritis.
Asthma.
Attention deficit.

B.
Bad breath.
Bites.
Bladder.
Bleeding.
Blisters.
Bloat.
Bad blood.

Blood poisoning.
Body odour.
Boils.
Bones.
Bone infections.
Bruises.
Bronchitis.
Broken wind.
Broodiness.
Burns.

C.
Cancers.
Car sickness.
Catarrh.
Cataract.
Centipede.
Chills.
Cholera.
Coccidiosis.
Colic.
Collapse.
Comb and wattles.
Concussion.
Conjunctivitis.
Constipation.
Cough.
Contortions.
Convulsions.
Cow-pox.
Cramp.
Cuts.

Cystitis.

D.
Dandruff.
Deafness.
Dying.
Depression.
Dehydration.
Diarrhoea.
Distemper.
Dizziness.

E.
Ears.
Eyes.
Electrocution.
Emphysema.
Epilepsy.
Excitement.
Exhaustion.
Eczema.

F.
Fatigue.
Fears.
Feathers always ruffled.
Feet.
Fever.
Fissures.
Fits.

Fireworks (fear of).
Fleas.
Fluid loss.
Food poisoning.
Foot rot.
Foreign bodies.
Frost Bite.
Fur Loss.

G.
Gait.
Gangrene.
Giddiness.
Glands.
Glanders.
Grief.
Growths.
Gums.

H.
Haemorrhoids.
Hairball.
Hayfever.
Head injury.
Head swelling.
Head black (birds).
Heart.
Head blow (near death).
Heatstroke.
Hernia.
Herpes.

Hiccoughs.
Homesickness (kennels).
Horsefly bites.
Hotspots.
Hysteria.

I.
Immune system.
Indigestion.
Indifference.
Infection.
Infertility.
Injury.
Interest gone.
Insomnia.
Itchy ears.
Itches.

J.
Jaundice.
Jerks and twitches.
Joint pain.

K.
Kennel cough.
Kidney.

L.
Lameness.

Leeches.
Lice on birds.
Lightning strike.
Liver.
Lung.
Lyme.

❧

M.
Mange.
Mastitis.
Milk fever.
Mouth ulcers.
Muscular dystrophy.

❧

N.
Nausea.
Nervousness.
Newcastle disease.
Nipples.
Noise sensitivity.
Nose.

❧

O.
Oil covered and cleaned.
Operations (surgery).
Orchitis.

❧

P.
Pain.

Panic.
Paralysis.
Parasites.
Parvo virus.
Piles.
Poisoning.
Pox.
Pneumonia.
Pregnancy (false).
Prolapse.

R.
Rabies.
Rage.
Respiratory disease.
CRD.
Restlessness.
Rheumatism.
Ring.
Ringworm.
Rubbing.
Rundown.

S.
Sadness.
Septicaemia.
Shock.
Skin (see eczema and mange).
Snakebite.
Sneezing.
Solitude.

Spasms.
Spinal injury.
Stiffness.
Stings.
Stinking body and discharges.
Storms.
Strangles.
Sunstroke.
Sulking (prolonged).
Surgery.
Swallowing.
Swelling.

T.
Teething.
Terror (see panic, fear).
Tetanus.
Thunder.
Tongue.
Touch.
Travel sickness.
Trembling.
Tuberculosis.
Tumours.
Twitches.
Typhoid.

U.
Ulcers on skin.
Umbilical infection.
Unconsciousness.

Urinary problems.

᠁

V.
Vaccinosis.
Vomitting.

᠁

W.
Warts.
Wax in ears.
Weakness.
Wheezing, no air.
Wounds.
Worms.

᠁

Y.
Yawning.

Index of Remedies in the Materia Medica.

B.
Bacc.
Baryta c.
Bapt.
Bell.
Bellis.
Berb vul.
Beryl m.
Bor.
Both.
Bov.
Bry.
Bufo.

C.
Cactus.
Calad.
Calc carb.
Calc fluor.
Calc phos.
Calc sulph.
Calend.
Cann ind.
Cann sat.
Canth.
Carbo veg.
Carot.
Caust.
Chamo.
Chel.
China.
Choles.

Cic vir.
Cim rac.
Cine.
Clem.
Coca.
Coccid fowl.
Coccus cacti.
Coffea.
Collin.
Coloc.
Con mac.
Crot hor.
Cup met.

D.
Digit.
Dros.
Dulc.

E.
Echin.
Euph.

F.
Ferrum phos.

G.
Gels.
Glon.

Golon.
Graph.
Guaco.

༄

H.
Ham.
Hekla lava.
Hep sul.
Hist.
Hyos.
Hyper.
Hydroph.

༄

I.
Ignat.
Indigo.
Iod.
Ipecac.

༄

J.
Jabor (Pilo mic).

༄

K.
Kali bich.
Kali mur.
Kali phos.
Kali sulph.
Kreos.

༄

L.
Lach.
Lact ac.
Lath sat.
Ledum.
Lil tig.
Lob.
Lyco.
Lyssin.

M.
Mag phos.
Merc cor (hydrarge).
Merc viv.
Mille.
Mur ac.

N.
Naphth.
Nat mur.
Nit ac.
Nux vom.

O.
Onos.
Opium.

P.
Passiflora.

Petrol.
Phos.
Phos ac.
Pic ac.
Phyto.
Pilo mic (see Jaborandi).
Plumb m.
Podo.
Psor.
Puls.
Pyro.

R.
Ranunc.
Rescue r.
Rhod.
Rhus tox.
Ruta g.

S.
Sabad.
Sabina.
Secale.
Sepia.
Sil.
Sinaps nig.
Spig.
Spong tost.
Squilla.
Stann met.
Staph.

Stramm.
Strepto.
Strych.
Sulph.
Symph.

❧

T.
Tabac.
Tarent hisp.
Tell.
Teuc.
Therid cur.
Thuja.
Trill pen.
Tuber.
Typhoid.

❧

U.
Urt u.

❧

V.
Vario.
Ver alb.
Vesp crab.

❧

Y.
Yohimb.

❧

Z
Zinc met.
Zing.

For.
Gringo, Pukkie, Bullet, Barry, Mrs Tego, Squeak, Stripe, Valentine, Melody, Caesar, Bathmat, Donna, Lupa, Muffin, Kelly, Bouvie, Pickle and Pepper the twin Schipperkes, Ross, Kumi and all the others.

I.
Vis Medicatrix Naturae.

This refers to the natural healing power within any body. It is the ability to recognise and repel invaders and repair damage caused by any source. Sometimes this ability can be impaired to various degrees. It is difficult to fully define where disease begins and ends, but when the natural healing powers are not properly functional, then a state of disease is presumed to exist.

There are two major forms of medicine available to assist the body in regaining its natural powers. The one is the medicine of contraries, e.g. where to medicate for pain, a pain-killer is administered. The other is the medicine of Similars, where a substance which causes the same symptoms in a healthy patient, as the patient to be treated exhibits, is administered in miniscule form, and it jogs the body into repelling the problem. The dose is so infinitesimal that not even one single atom is administered, only the nuclear imprint of it, with the substance diluted millions of times. A complete atom might kill the patient at times, since the substances used are sometimes deadly poisonous in undiluted form. However, in diluted form they are completely harmless, and have no effect whatsoever on a healthy body.

Homeopathy is based on the administration of the Simillimum, or the Similar, and is totally safe with no side-effects. Once the Vis Medicatrix Naturae has been activated, the body heals all its own problems without further assistance. Naturally this makes very little money for the remedy manufacturers, and would put many orthodox medicine manufacturers out of business, so consequently the orthodox establishment sometimes goes to extreme lengths to try to discredit homeopathy. Imagine a manufacturer of childrens' medicines (among others in a huge range of products), which sells eighty million doses per day, making an average of one dollar per dose, per day for many years, per child. Considering a homeopathic dose might cure the problem, you can imagine what gigantic stakes are really at play here. Of course this is not the case with all manufacturers nor all orthodox medicines, but I am sure you can see the principle here. Homeopathy can not cause depressions, suicidal tendencies and other side-effects. It also cannot cure many potentially fatal diseases that orthodox medicine can treat with various invasive techniques and emergency procedures, blood transfusions, x-rays and similar. Assess the strength of your patient's Vis Medicatrix Naturae (people can be very good at assessing their patient's Vital Force), and decide which path to follow. Hopefully this book will provide you with some assistance in the choice of treatment of animals and birds, and possibly even humans.

Hippocrates, the famous Greek physician, taught that medicines merely created the correct conditions for the individual's natural healing power, the Vis Medicatrix Naturae, to restore the balance of the system, and enable it to remove the symptoms of illness.

The Vis Medicatrix Naturae is inextricably interwoven with the concept of the Vital Force, the activation of which, by the administration of homeopathic remedies, leads to recovery from various ills and injuries. The natural healing power within the person, is powered by the Vital Force, or "chi" or "prana", which is an urgent, driven, powerful energy, sometimes dormant and sometimes active. Specially trained people can summon or activate this force at will. The natural healing power is also evidenced in ways which show its presence, other than in healing. For instance a small woman is suddenly able to carry a heavy child at a run for a long distance to escape danger. Sometimes this natural healing power is activated by external forces, and other times by the system itself, but when it is not in action as it should be, it can be stimulated into action by homeopathic remedies. Also by focus and concentration, self-hypnosis, hypnosis, meditation, acupuncture and yoga, and other complementary systems, the Vital force or natural healing powers can be jolted into curing illnesses and other problems. It is something akin to a supercharger of bodily abilities and mental fortitude.

The Vis Medicatrix Naturae is not visible to the eye, except in its manifestations of energy, healing etc in a person, and is in itself a major energy field. It is also present in animals, birds, fish, plants, trees and living entities.

Some current speculation regards the natural healing power as a possible bioplasm of ionised particles, held in proximity to each other by energy. It is thought to affect growth and development as it effects repairs on the system. It may be an energy double of the physical body, tightly connected, and interlaced with all its aspects. Its stimulation leads to recovery from illness and injury. The healing force effects changes in mind, body and emotions.

The healing power of the body, is an inherent ability to establish, maintain and restore good health. Nature heals through the response of the Vis Medicatrix Naturae, which is an ordered and intelligent process. The homeopath's remedy facilitates and augments this process, to act and identify and remove obstacles to health and recovery, and to support the creation of a healthy internal and external environment.

First described in western medicine by Hippocrates, the Vis Medicatrix Naturae, is also referred to as "chi" in Chinese Medicine, "prana" in Ayurveda, and "Vital Force" in homeopathy. When alive, the Vis Medicatrix Naturae enables humans and other living beings to resist entropy and decay, unlike inanimate objects that are not subject to these effects at the same rapid rate that living beings are. Creating treatment plans that harness the healing power of nature, that incorporate dietary and lifestyle improvements, that employ the least invasive, least harmful and most effective therapies, is the art, the heart and the essence of homeopathic medicine.

2.

The History Of Homeopathy, With Reference To "China", Or Cinchona Officinalis, A Remedy.

ॐ

"China" has great historical significance, and is inextricably linked with Dr Samuel Hahnemann, in the context of the formation of modern homeopathy. An Edinburgh teacher, physician and chemist, wrote a book entitled "A Treatise on Materia Medica". The teacher's name was Dr William Cullen, and he lived from 1710 to 1790. The book included an essay on Peruvian bark, or Cinchona, which homeopaths call "China", from which quinine, the treatment for malaria, is derived. Cullen attributed Cinchona's quality of curing malaria, with its symptoms of periodic fever, sweating and palpitations, to its bitterness (describing a "tonic" action on the stomach). Hahnemann was not taken in by this explanation, being aware of more astringent medicines which did not cure malaria, and decided to test the remedy on himself. This he did by boiling up the bark of Cinchona Officionalis, and drinking the noxious fluid for several days, after which he succumbed to his famous acute bout of malarial-like symptoms.

In a letter, he described exactly what symptoms the remedy caused in himself, being among other symptoms, a coldness creeping in from the extremities, languidness, palpitations, anxiety and trembling, pulsation in the head, then all the symptoms of a general fever, and these occurred every time he dosed himself, and lasted for two or three hours. So in fact, Hahnemann showed that the remedy produced in himself, all the symptoms of malaria, which it was known to cure. In turn, he could speculate that because Cinchona produced the symptoms of malaria in a normal, healthy human being, that was why it cured malaria, and therefore any substance which produced the symptoms of any disease in a normal, healthy human being, might very well cure that disease. This was the basis, the founding principle, of modern homeopathy.

As Hahnemann developed his investigations, he was able to observe the symptoms any substance produced on a normal healthy person, and so discover the healing properties of that substance. The remedy then is shown to act on that part of the body which it most resembles. This procedure was called "proving", or testing a remedy.

The basic assumption until that time, and still prevalent in some forms of medical practice, was that if the body produced a symptom, then the appropriate medicine would be the antidote to that symptom. As an example, constipation would be treated with laxatives. Hippocrates had written long ago, about the medicine of "similars", which involved treating the symptom with a remedy which caused the same symptom in a healthy person. Hahnemann simply confirmed this principle, called the "similia similibus curentur" (let like be cured with like). This principle became the first law of the system of healing called homeopathy, from the Greek, meaning similar (homeo) and pathos (disease). The name differentiated it from orthodox medicine, called "allopathy", from allo (opposite) and pathy (suffering).

Hahnemann, as a result of his China experiments or provings, opened his new medical practice with a different way of prescribing. As he wrote, he noted three forms of curing, the first being the removal of the causes of the malady, being preventative treatment, and secondly there is the treating with opposites as in allopathic medicine, and finally there is the treating with the similia similibus, which means treating a disease with the medicine which excites similar symptoms in healthy people. (1796).

During the next six years, Hahnemann conducted numerous provings on friends and family, and also studied accounts of the symptoms of victims of accidental poisonings. Finally when he set up his medical practice, he only sought the simillimum, or similar, the remedy which most matched the symptoms of his patients, or was most similar, as that is what cures them. He was ridiculed by the establishment but stuck to his guns and proved them all wrong.

Some famous homeopathic names and a little bit of history.

To name just a few, Dr. James Tyler Kent, MD (1849-1910), Dr.Constantine Hering, MD (1800-1880), and Dr. Carrol Dunhum, MD (1828-1877) from USA, Dr. Richard Hughes, MD (1836-1902), and Dr. John Henry Clarke, MD (1853-1931) from UK, Dr. Carl Von Boenninghausen, MD(1785-1864) from Netherlands, Dr. Rajendra Lal Dutt, MD

(1818-1889), Dr. Mahendra Lal Sircar, MD (1833-1904), and Dr. Pratap Muzumdar, MD from India, are some of the other eminent homeopaths who have contributed to homeopathy with their research, new remedies and books. Most of these doctors were successful allopaths who became homeopaths after they/their family members were cured through the use of homeopathy after experiencing long-term health problems.

Despite significant antagonism from medical manufacturers and the orthodox medical profession, homeopathy has survived and is growing strongly. Homeopathy has attracted support from many of the most respected members of society including Mahatma Gandhi, William Cullen Bryant, the famous journalist, and Britain's Royal family since the 1830s. You only have to see how long-lived and healthy the Royal Family is, to draw your own conclusions about homeopathy. The most significant reason why homeopathy has developed immense popularity is its success in treating the various infectious epidemic diseases that raged throughout America and Europe during the 1800s. Statistics indicate that the death rates in homeopathic hospitals from these epidemics were often one-half to as little as one-eighth of those in orthodox medical hospitals. The same result was found on battlefields, where wounded men had an extraordinary rate of recovery when treated homeopathically.

Homeopathy is very popular in Europe, the USA, Asia (especially in India), Sri Lanka and Pakistan. It is also widely practiced in Brazil, Mexico, Greece, Belgium, Italy, Spain, Australia, South Africa, Nigeria, and the former Soviet Union.

In a cursory look at one hundred and ten obituaries

of famous homeopaths, one homeopath found that the average age at death was eighty-four. This goes back many years.

3.
The Nature of Homeopathy.

◆

Definition of Homeopathy.

◆

Homeopathy is a system of medicine based on the principle of treating like with like. Its name derives from the Greek words "homoios" (like) and "pathos" (suffering). It is designed to restore the human being to a state of equilibrium, and therefore health, by treating the causes of illness, acute and chronic disease, accidents, befallments and acute mistunements, traumas, emotional and mental disturbances, rather than symptoms. By the administration of a pathogenic substance, which in itself produces the same symptoms in a healthy person, as the patient has, the organism (human being usually) is "kickstarted" into curing itself. Homeopathy is characterised by this principle, which is termed the "similia law" or "law of similars".

Homeopathy is holistic in nature, treating the constitution, or whole person, rather than symptoms in isolation. Remedies used are the tiniest possible doses of natural substances, like plants, animals, insects and minerals. Homeopathy frees patients from disease symptoms, and restores inner harmony, improving energy, work, relationships and life. Homeopathy stimulates the

Vital Force within the patient, which regulates and repairs and heals the system.

❧

The two main principles of homeopathy.

❧

a) The first principle (Law of Similars) initially states that every active substance that acts on the functions of the body provokes a set of symptoms characteristic to that substance in a healthy, sensitive body. An example of this is coffee, which causes an acceleration of the heart rate, increased urine output, nervous excitation, insomnia and a heightening of the senses. Now the principle states that any substance which can make you ill can also cure you. If it can produce the symptoms of the disease in a healthy body, then it can also cure those symptoms in a sick body.

Every diseased body exhibits a range of symptoms characteristic to that illness. An example of this is mental overexertion, which produces a heightened heart rate, insomnia, excitability, a racing mind, increased sensitivity to noise or light and touch.

These two phenomena are the basics used to identify a cure, which will be demonstrated by the disappearance of the symptoms, brought about by the prescription of a low or infinitesimal dose of a substance that would produce similar symptoms in a healthy person. Therefore COFFEA in homeopathic dose, would cure the above patient. This is a demonstration of the Law of Similars, being the principle of "let like be treated by like", or similia similibus curentur. The symptom profile must always be matched with the remedy profile, as one is treating the patient, not the disease. Each patient will probably demonstrate some different symptom profiles for the same disease, and so will not necessarily be treated with the same remedy as everyone else, and each patient should be treated as an individual, needing individualised treatment, rather than being grouped by disease for a remedy e.g. giving everyone with a sore throat the same remedy (which would be homeopathically wrong but perhaps correct for orthodox medicine). Unless the Law of Similars is correctly applied, the treatment will be worthless.

b) The second principle is the Law of Potentised Remedies. Extreme dilution enhances the curative properties of a substance, while eliminating side-effects. Furthermore, in conventional medicine, as the concentration is decreased, so the medicine becomes less effective (potent), until a point is reached where it stops working, whereas in homeopathic medicine with each dilution (and succussion, or violent shake) it gains in potency, and this is the basis of homeopathic Potentised Remedies. This is what separates homeopathy from orthodox medicine, and upsets those rigid minds of critics who cannot conceive of something beyond their preconceptions. In homeopathy the energy levels present in the remedies are what promote the cure, and not the actual amount of the substance. As all remedies have many facets, and can produce various symptoms in healthy people, it is possible and preferable to prescribe only a single correct remedy at a time. By doing this its precise effect can be observed, and the homeopath can proceed further with other remedies for stubborn or newly-emerging other symptoms. Furthermore, it is commonly felt that the smallest possible dose required to nudge the healing process into action, is the best. This is in keeping with the highly diluted and therefore highly potentised homeopathic remedy that homeopaths use.

The term, "the similar".

❧

The "similar" refers to the homeopathic remedy, which when administered to a healthy body, will cause that body to exhibit the same symptoms as the patient is experiencing. The appropriate use of processed substances similar to the disease, can restore a sick body to a state of balance, and therefore health. Diseases are therefore shown to succumb to substances which cause a similar ailment, hence the word "similar" to describe each substance. Hahnemann suggested that this is because nature will not allow two similar diseases to exist in the body at the same time, so the newly introduced one will push the old one out. Each patient does not respond to a "similar" in the same way as every other patient, and because each patient exhibits a different response, an entire "symptom picture" of each patient needs to be found, so that the selected "similar" will match the patient's individual needs in as many ways as possible, and not simply become a general hit-or-miss remedy. A "similar" may be identified by careful use of a Materia Medica, once the patient's profile has been established. A good Materia Medica lists all symptoms a substance may cause in a healthy person, and therefore a study of substances to find one which most perfectly matches the patient's symptoms, will expose the closest "similar" for appropriate administration.

A "similar" should be selected on the basis of causing similar symptoms (in a healthy body), to the patient's symptoms, in as many fields as possible. These include characteristics (e.g. fidgets), general symptoms (like attitude, outlook, reactions to the disease and other matters of life), mentals (emotional makeup, fears, phobias, drives, introversions etc), modalities (all matters which aggravate or ameliorate the situation, like weather, season, body position, time of day, eating, water, keeping still, and numerous others), likes and dislikes (cravings and aversions), physical characteristics (expression, walk, posture, appearance, skin, hair etc), disease tendencies of the past and present, family history (reason for, and time of deaths), patient's history (trauma etc), emotional tendencies such as doubt, agoraphobia etc.). The better the remedy matches the patient profile the more effectively it will cure the patient. A homeopath should always seek the most perfect, or closest "similar", starting with the mentals, then going on to the reactions to the world, then cravings and aversions and then the particulars to that patient's body, broadly speaking (Kent).

The above information is sometimes termed differently, and Hahnemann, the great German physician, termed all the patient information the "symptom picture". The symptoms induced in healthy people by substances (drugs), he called the "drug picture". The more similar the "symptom picture" and the "drug picture" are, the more likely the treatment is to be successful, and the stronger the likelihood that the remedy and the disease will cancel each other out. It is always necessary to find the patient's symptoms first, before matching them to different remedies so as to find the most appropriate one.

4.
The Arndt-Shultz Law.

This Law states that weak stimuli slightly accelerate the Vital Force, middle strong stimuli raise it a little, strong ones suppress it and very strong ones halt it altogether. This is the principle behind the administration of an infinitesimal dose of homeopathic remedy, to patients. The principle also applies to animals, insects and other living organisms, such as yeast, where one can observe that every stimulus on a living cell elicits an activity which is inversely proportional to the intensity of the stimulus. The weaker or more diluted a homeopathic remedy is, the stronger will be its effect upon a patient. The least effective dilutions such as 6X (6x10) are not nearly as deep-acting on the entire system as for examples LM (50x1000) dilutions, or the serially diluted Bach remedies which are diluted and succussed thousands of times to have a powerful effect upon the mind and body of patients.

The more diluted (or "weak") they are the greater is their effect, so demonstrating the Arndt-Shultz Law.

A term used in regard to this Law is "Hormesis". The word "hormesis" is derived from the Greek word "hormaein" which means "to excite". It has long been known that many popular substances such as alcohol and caffeine have mild stimulating effects in low doses but are detrimental or even lethal in high doses. In the early 1940s C. Southam and a co-worker J. Erlish found that despite the fact that high concentrations of Oak bark extract inhibited fungi growth in sample fungi, low doses of this agent stimulated fungi growth. In regards to radiation treatment of cancers, it has been suggested by some researchers that lower radiation frequencies should be used than are presently being used, as they might be more effective.

Fundamentally, certain treatments can poison and/or kill patients when administered to patients in pure form, but when they are diluted or reduced sufficiently to not poison, then they may result in a self-recovery action from the patient. Effectiveness is therefore a function of concentration, in reverse. Excessive, increasing concentration causes the treatment to be reflected by the constitution of the patient, ever-more completely. This principle enables homeopaths to use the most toxic substances (snake poison, deadly plants, chemicals etc) as healing remedies, as they are assimilated when in potentised form (serially diluted and succussed, which is in essence a violent shaking).

The "Concept of Potency" and the meaning of "Potency Number".

Substances can be diluted and succussed to potentise remedies, which become more effective (potent) with each dilution. Potency numbers reflect how many times the mother tincture has been succussed not just diluted, with 30C being popular but extending to LM times and more.

5.
Naming The Disease, Or Not?

Each substance tested produces a whole set of signs, which result in a symptom picture, or remedy picture. These consist of a list of sensations, thought patterns, physical and mental problems. When a body gets sick or finds itself in a condition of disease, then the body presents a symptom picture too, which will correspond with the symptom picture of a homeopathic remedy. The challenge of homeopathy, is to seek out the complete symptom picture of the patient, and find the exact, or closest match among the remedy pictures. This match will cure the disease. Orthodox medicine, with its desperation to neatly box all phenomena into sterile packages, will label the disease as something, imagining that it stands alone and is identical in all bodies. It will also provide a standard treatment for all patients diagnosed with that illness.

Homeopathy, on the other hand, does not diagnose a named illness but takes cognisance of the complete patient picture, including all ascertainable symptoms, and prescribes the closest matching remedy. The secret to the most effective remedy is for the homeopath to find all the information he needs and to correctly do the matching. This can be extremely difficult with humans, or children, but is more difficult with animals who cannot provide the information you need. For instance a guinea-pig cannot tell you how restless he is at night, or that he is over-producing saliva, or that his limbs ache before storms, or that he keeps fantasising that other guinea-pigs are victimising him. He can also not describe the development of his disease, nor even tell you about the thistles he ate to try to cure himself. The homeopath is faced with what he can see, and what he can interpret from watching the animal, and what he can learn from the owners. Anything that has changed in the animal's pattern, should be regarded as relevant. A five minute glance is not likely to deliver much quality information to the homeopath, who needs to spend time with the animal, assessing the moods, fears, pains, digestive situation and everything else. It takes the author around two hours to even break the ice with human patients and can take longer with animals.

However, in the case of first response treatment, or being in a hurry, or needing to treat a symptom as rapidly as possible to preserve life and ease pain, then the presenting symptom can be looked at and prescribed for, in isolation.

The list which appears later in this book is based on this kind of situation. It is a quick response guide to anyone needing to react to a situation, or without the wherewithal to properly investigate the pictures. After the first reaction, it would be as well to seek the more appropriate remedies. The guide does point you in the right direction and the suggested remedies can form the basis of a more thorough investigation.

6.
The Complete Organism, Iatrogenisis And Vaccinosis.

કે

As can be seen, homeopathy takes cognisance of the complete organism and all its symptoms and manifestations. It is naturopathic in character and should be combined with a healthy general approach to life. Naturopathic Medicine, a primary health-care system, treats health conditions by utilizing the body's inherent ability to heal. Naturopathic physicians aid the healing process by incorporating a variety of alternative methods based on the patient's individual needs — nutrition, herbal medicine, homeopathic medicine and oriental medicine. Diet, lifestyle, work and personal history are all considered when determining regimen. Traditionally homeopathy tends to rely more on its own abilities, but in the author's view it should be combined with a healthy diet, adequate rest, minimum stress and some exercise.

Every year numerous new orthodox medicines appear, and are hailed as the new wonder drugs, making millions for their manufacturers and sellers. If they alleviate a symptom of something, they are widely acclaimed, and then are soon forgotten in the mists of time with all the other drugs. Within a few years side-effects start to show, and the products are withdrawn quietly. This has given rise to a host of new disease called "iatrogenic diseases", which are diseases caused by medicines, from the Greek word "iatros" meaning medicine. In other words, patience, tender loving care and compassion have been replaced by incompletely tested drugs which are pumped into bodies as fast as possible with the intention of making as much money as possible.

There are growing numbers of articles appearing, which comment on the ever-increasing chronic ill health plaguing Western pets. Their immune systems are suffering breakdown, there is a big discrepancy between their lifespans now and what they used to be, skin and ear allergies proliferate, digestive disorders are common, thyroid, adrenal and pancreatic disorders abound, spleens rupture, seizures are common, gums and teeth have problems, there is degenerative arthritis, kidney and liver failure and cancer. This all stretches across all breeds of all sexes. In addition there are record numbers of emotional and behavioural problems, nervous disorders and attention deficiency problems. Much of this may be attributed to the overuse of multiple vaccines and toxin-filled, under-nutritious commercial pet foods. Add to this the many diseases which have never been cured, but only suppressed by anti-biotics, drugs and cortisone, and you see our pets are in a bad way.

In the case of vaccinations, chemically killed viruses and bacteria are injected directly into the body, flooding the blood with their particles. Long term results range from auto-immune and life-threatening crises, to appalling skin allergies which severely reduce the quality of life of the sufferers. A growing body of thought has found that booster vaccinations are completely unnecessary, because of their side-effects. These side-effects can be treated homeopathically...see Vaccinosis in the guide.

Dr. Chambreau, the renowned veterinary homeopath, has commented that dogs in Germany, which have only one vaccination and no boosters, live to around six years longer than those in the UK and USA, which are subjected to boosters. Canadian dogs also live around six years longer, according to another source. Homeopathic treatment should be used rather than vaccinations.

7.
It Is Better To Maintain Good Health Than To Treat Diseases.

People who do not know which factors are bad for animal health, can easily find out. They are virtually the same as those that are bad for human health. Homeopathy works best on a body which is not abused with toxins, is correctly fed, adequately rested and free of excess stress and worry. It strengthens the immune system, prevents illnesses from occurring before they happen, makes bodies resistant to most epidemics, and lessens the chances of latent problems suddenly emerging in later life. A body in full good health keeps itself free of diseases, and full of energy and good cheer. Constitutional remedies help a great deal in this regard, causing the entire system to be robust and disease resistant.

Diseases which have been suppressed but not cured, can result in many later emergences of symptoms. For instance, a body might suffer from a constantly running nose, which is treated only with sprays and other symptomatic medications, and later becomes sinus and post-nasal drip, and then asthma, and when only treated as asthma, develops into arthritis, early ageing symptoms, and finally boils and eczema, followed by an early, unpleasant death. Correct building up of the entire system, with constitutional remedies (see later), can prevent the spread of disease from the beginning. However, if a homeopath is consulted at an intermediate stage, he might be able to reverse the trend, and peel away the layers of disease, to expose and free the healthy body underneath. However, if permanent damage has already occurred, it may be too late.

The unhealthy topic of manufactured and toxic foods has already been touched on. Remember it is also necessary for animals to enjoy lots of exercise. They, like you, are designed with a functional body which thrives on physical activity. Do not cage animals in small areas, and ensure that domestic ones have plenty of exercise. The scope of this book does not cover this topic in more detail.

Human beings can retain an exceptional level of health by regularly doing QiGong, a system of exercises which stretch each part of the body, and include deep, regular breathing. This results in complete oxygenation of the body, which assists good health. While it is not possible to teach QiGong to animals, they must be allowed the opportunity to exercise themselves properly.

8.
The Immune System.

꙳

Micro-organisms from the environment constantly attack your animals. Animals defend themselves from these frequently deadly attacks, by using their immune systems. Complex and violent wars to the death are waged, until one or the other loses, and is killed. Allopathic drugs try to attack these micro-organisms, but homeopathic remedies feed and strengthen the immune system so that it can effectively fight the battle on its own.

Immune systems grow and develop inside babies before they are born. When an attack takes place, a host of chemical messages are activated, like dispatch riders in an army, carrying information to the troops, which rush out and attack viciously. After the battle, the troops never leave, but remain there on standby, ready to deal with a similar attack at any time in the future.

Attacks are mainly carried out by parasites, fungi, protozoa (e.g. malaria), bacteria and viruses, which cause infectious diseases. The body's first line of defence is the skin, and the mucous membranes. These keep out most infections. Should they breach these defences, they will encounter a very effective system in place underneath them. This is called the immune system and the study of this is termed "immunology".

The immune system in a healthy body is ready at all

times, and will act at once to kill or immobilize any invaders. However, there are two types of immunity, the one being passive immunity, which we are born with, and the other being acquired immunity which we develop when we come into contact with nasty viruses or bacteria. After each response, a memory remains, which enables the system to instantly respond when faced with the same attack at any time in the future. This is good, because it can take the body a long time to react effectively against some attacks, and if it takes too long the patient dies. Vaccinations work on this principle, establishing this memory so a body can react rapidly in the future to a similar attack. Millions of lives are saved this way. It is only when too many vaccinations take place that danger occurs.

9.
Acute And Chronic Conditions.

An acute condition comes on quickly and often departs quickly. It can be caused by infection or temporary imbalance of the system, or stress, injury, overexertion etc. Infections causing acute conditions can be colds, coughs or bacterial or viral infections. Acute also refers to bruising, bleeding, convulsions or loss of consciousness. In acute conditions that the homeopath cannot cope with, a doctor should be called. Orthodox medicine has symptom drugs for acute conditions, such as anti-spasm, anti-coagulant, stings, and so on. Acute conditions are new and recent, not deep-seated, and sometimes clear on their own. Some can be fatal, such as meningitis, nephritis or pneumonia. Acute diseases have the distinct phases of incubation (no symptoms), acute phase (the symptoms surface), and the convalescent phase showing strong improvement. Home remedies ease the pain and speed up recovery in many acute illnesses such as food poisoning, 'flu and childrens' illnesses, ensuring there are no complications.

Acute states are departures from the usual state and can be physical or mental/emotional.

A chronic condition is quite different, showing a history of various complaints, with deep underlying causes, recurrences, lowered vitality and steadily declining general health. People feel unwell yet medical tests reveal nothing. The origins may be chronic diseases. Chronic diseases mistune the living organism with small unnoticed beginnings, and the state of health declines, steadily until death. The Vital Force is unable to stop this as it increases mistunement, leading to final destruction of the organism.

There is an idea, incorrect, among certain people, that the word "acute" refers to the sharpness or degree of severity of a complaint. This is not accurate, as a chronic complaint may be much more painful or severe than an acute one, in some instances.

Unlike acute diseases, a chronic disease does not take a predictable course, and one cannot say how long it will last. It can even stem from the complications following an acute disease. Examples of chronic disease are heart problems, cancer and mental illness. Some may be caused by chemicals in food and in the air, overuse of orthodox medicines (e.g. painkillers) and general environmental pollution....chemical, noise, too many people etc.

An acute illness may be infectious so the patient may need to keep away from other people. In some cases only rest may be needed for people to recover, or perhaps, relaxation, fresh air, good food and some pampering. A chronic state is probably not infectious and will probably become worse irrespective of rest or diet and pampering. Acute cases can be caused by simple exhaustion and being run down, but chronic ones are deep-seated, arising from infection or miasms passed down from previous generations.

People suffering from acute conditions can usually pinpoint the problem e.g. a very sore joint, or a sore throat, while in chronic cases the patient probably suffers from a host of different symptoms (seemingly unrelated as far as the patient is concerned). Treatment for acute symptoms is usually specific and may be aimed at soft tissue, with short-lasting low potency remedies. Chronic conditions may need years of treatment or a long time to recover, with the use of high potency remedies, or constitutional remedies.

Acute conditions may require frequent taking of remedies even down to every fifteen minutes or so in extremis (e.g. head injury) while chronic treatments may require a single remedy taken once, which acts for months or years. Acute conditions may clear very rapidly, perhaps even within the hour, while chronic ones may take years.

It is very simple to repertorise for an acute condition as it often is a case of single symptom repertorising, but chronic conditions may require many hours of sleuthing and hard work to identify symptoms, construct a good symptom picture, and then match it to remedies to try to find the most complete match.

Trauma rooms and outpatient's departments in hospitals, usually deal with acute situations, like falls down steps. Chronic ones have gone on for a long time and do not call for sudden intervention, like oxygen, operations, pain killers, sedatives etc, except at the end.

There are certain acute conditions which require urgent medical attention and where a doctor should be consulted. Homeopaths can make these situations more comfortable, but should not attempt to deal with them. They are neck and back injuries, chest and abdominal wounds, protruding or broken bones, burns that are not small, cyanosis (turning blue), chest pains, unconsciousness, severe head injury, seizures, difficulty in breathing, shock for more than an hour, bleeding more than just a little bit. In chronic conditions there is not this sudden trauma, but a slow insidious ingress of problems over a long period, perhaps decades.

Some common acute situations are injuries, food poisoning, insect or snake or dog bites, burns or scalds, gastro-intestinal problems, cuts and abrasions. There are quite different to chronic situations like cancers, rheumatism, arthritis etc.

One source says a rule of thumb for determining whether a condition is acute or chronic, is whether it arrives and clears within six months or not. Perhaps this is too simplistic a model.

10.
Fundamental Disease.

This concept originates with the possibility that all manifestations of illness (symptoms) are merely indicators of a fundamental disease within the system. This disease affects, from within, the body and mind of the sufferer. The subtle body is affected and unable to tune all the aspects of the Vital Force adequately, so as to ensure vibrant good health. Because of this mistunement, different problems and symptoms appear at different times. The symptoms are an indicator of the fundamental disease.

Symptoms are not seen in isolation, as with orthodox medicine, but can be collected and listed, and will point to the fundamental cause of them all. Fundamental diseases collect in the body sometimes, like walled off capsules, emerging from time to time when the Vital Force, weakened by the fundamental disease, is not able to maintain the walls adequately. Sometimes these manifestations are described as rings (like in an onion), with each ring being a burned out or suppressed disease, waiting to show a symptom, when the fundamental disease weakens the Vital Force sufficiently. They can be caused by, or brought into existence by various things such as drugs or antibiotics (suppression) or by trauma, mental or emotional (death, stress) or physical causes (motor accident). Each one leaves a residue or imprint. In a healthy body they may never emerge again, but in a weakened one they may emerge in different forms from time to time. A wart, for instance, when cut off, may cause other symptoms to emerge, such as asthma, as they could all be caused by the same fundamental disease. Suppression or removing of a symptom (which the system is using as a valve to cope with the disease) may increase the internal pressure, resulting in the emergence of other symptoms. It may be better to treat the fundamental disease with constitutional remedies, than to treat local symptoms and leave the fundamental disease untouched and active. Activity on individual symptoms, may activate or stimulate the fundamental disease.

Ultimately, a very complicated interaction among the layers of disease, may arise from interference with individual symptoms, resulting in multi-system chronic disease. A whole range of symptoms may then simultaneously arise, and defy all efforts to deal with them. An example might be the arthritis, skin problems and emotional changes of rheumatoid arthritis, or otherwise catarrh, migraine and colitis.

Hahnemann found that the disposition of a patient was a decidedly characteristic symptom which should chiefly determine the selection of a homeopathic remedy. He also noted that a complete picture of an individual required an understanding of the primary, latent and secondary states of fundamental miasms. In his early days he noted that some patients responded not at all, or less and less, to remedies, indicating that a fundamental disease was operating and perhaps causing all the chronic symptoms. For twelve years he sought the fundamental cause of the symptoms which plagued some patients, and in various great works he concluded that chronic miasms could be responsible. One can have a number of miasms all contributing to disease and various symptoms, and they can be a fundamental cause, and also an obstruction to remedies. In short, they form a sort of fundamental disease, or set of diseases, within patients suffering from chronic diseases.

In order to discover a fundamental cause, whether it be a miasm or not, the investigation should include all ascertainable information about the physical state of the patient, their moral and intellectual character, occupation, mode of living and habits, social and domestic relations, age, sexual function and everything else. Since a fundamental disease will affect all of this, it can also cause various symptoms.

Fundamental diseases can be slow, insidious, with a gradual onset and slow progression. Complex pathologies result, and premature old age and death follow. They damage the Vital Force, the immune system, and the constitution.

So while it may not be completely possible to describe what a fundamental disease really is, the totality of symptoms can make us aware of its existence, and point to appropriate remedies. This has been a very brief description of the fundamental disease and fundamental cause.

II.
Best Potency To Use In Acute Prescribing, For The Beginner.

In acute prescribing, the beginner might be best advised to stick to low potencies, until he is quite well experienced. Low potencies work well on localised problems, from pain (dentist, sprains) to mood problems (anxiety), can be administered in quick succession if symptoms re-occur, and act fast and satisfyingly. They only remain in the system briefly and do not work much on the mentals/emotionals, as do the higher potencies which may function for months and exert influence on the mind. Acute conditions should be viewed by the beginner as being local and superficial.

Acute conditions can develop into chronic ones, each forming a new ring in the onion ring model. Beginners can treat each layer using low potencies, as each layer's symptoms when exposed by removal of a more recent layer, can be seen as acute symptoms, and can be treated with low potencies. The outer layer is always the most recent one.

In cases of structural damage, low potencies should be used, and the problem should be regarded as acute eg arthritic pains in the finger joints (possibly Rhus tox 6C or up to 30C according to different sources). The low potency will alleviate the pain in the manner of a local anaesthetic. 200C etc is not called for in these cases, although the problem is chronic and has been there for years.

As newly qualified homeopaths learn, they come to identify constitutional remedies, but early on this may prove exceedingly difficult to do. Because of this the symptoms should be tackled individually with low potencies, working from the latest backwards. In this way each acute layer can be peeled off as soon as it appears, exposing the previous symptoms in the next layer, which then seem acute, until finally the constitutional remedy can be spotted, no longer concealed by constantly emerging and changing acute symptoms.

High potencies have a greater effect on the whole person, including the emotional sphere and stay in the system longer. High potencies used by a beginner in treating acute symptoms may result in great discomfort and unwanted emotional changes. Beginners should move from low to high potencies slowly and with care, keeping careful tabs on their effects. Higher potencies take much longer to act, and this should be born in mind, and also discussed with the patient.

A beginner should also understand that patients bringing animals with acute problems do not want to wait a long time for results. They want immediate cure from the remedy and may not grasp your explanations of waiting and suffering any longer, being allopathically programmed into the idea of a quickfix by a pill or injection. They want the quickest local surface reaction possible to gain faith in the homeopath, who may explain again, and move on to higher potencies. Patients want acute problems sorted out as quickly as possible. In well-established pathologies, there may be no noticeable improvement for the first three months of treatment with high potencies. Low potencies may alleviate the symptoms in less than an hour, on occasion.

As to the exact potency to use, perhaps each homeopath has a different opinion. Up to 30C could be seen as a low, or medium potency (the country one happens to be in also influences the labelling of potencies as high or low). A lecturer at a local college, in homeopathy, told me not to use anything lower than 30C in treating acute problems, and advised me never to use any lower potency. A pharmacist/homeopath on the South Coast told me she prescribes D6 (Kali sulph for a skin condition), and variously D3 to D60 for acute conditions. An Asian homeopath suggested I use 6C for all acute conditions, at first. Perhaps all of them would be suitable.

In a chronic case, as a rule of thumb, when would one use a low potency and when would one use a high potency?

As a rule of thumb, a low potency may be used for acute or surface symptoms, such as cuts or scrapes or coughs, which have come on suddenly. They include symptoms, usually accompanied by great pain, which need immediate attention which will have a rapid effect. Low potencies such as 6C or 12C, as examples, work fast and quickly depart from the system, so can be administered again, perhaps even half-hourly, and up to a maximum of ten doses, then eight hours apart, for a maximum of three days. Burns, back injuries, earache, cystitis etc may respond well to low potencies, which act on soft tissue, such as muscle and skin, and can ease pain, shock and bleeding.

A high potency is slower acting and works on the mentals/emotionals, later having a spin-off effect on physical symptoms, or sometimes working on them at the same time. High potency is used for long-standing or chronic symptoms, which have been in place for months, or even years or decades. There is no sudden great rush and some homeopaths prescribe only a single dose of the appropriate remedy, and then wait to watch its result. A 30C remedy for instance, could be taken every twelve hours for three days, or a 200C remedy once, followed a week later by 30C daily for three days. The theory is that the 200C will jolt the Vital Force into action, and the 30C will ensure that it remains active. Generally the stronger the mental/emotional symptoms, the higher the potency, and the stronger the physical symptoms, the lower the potency should be.

Once the Vital Force responds, the remedy must be stopped until there is no further action, when it can be started again. Care should be taken not to confuse acute with chronic symptoms.

Kent noted (see Dr. Bahtia: Shirleys-wellness-café. com) that when the simillimum is found, the remedy will act curatively in a series of potencies. If the remedy is only partially similar, it will act in one or two potencies and then the symptoms will change and a new remedy will be required. This does not necessarily help with which potency to start with in the question, but it tells us that different potencies are dependent upon varying factors, to be fully effective.

Pulford, in the same website as above, has a different idea of what high or low potencies may be, but also agrees that low is better for acute illness and high for chronic.

He comments that the low curative remedies range from 30C to CC (200th) potencies (considered high by some standards), and are especially useful for acute diseases which do not rely on nor are part of a deep chronic malady. The medium curative remedies, he notes, range from CC to 10M potencies in subacute cases all of which rest upon some deeper "dyscrasia". The higher potencies range from 10M up for chronic curable diseases.

There are various views, supporting the principle that high potencies will cure both acute and chronic disease (if the simillimum is right), but that low potencies will only cure acute illnesses, although some writers say that low potencies will eventually act upon chronic illnesses after a long time. There is also a belief among some homeopaths, that high potencies will act faster and more effectively on acute problems than low potencies will. I have even found the idea that any potency will eventually act as a cure provided the simillimum is right.

When starting a remedy, it might be advisable, in some views, to start low and then work our way up, like music going up the harmonious scale. Here are some of the considerations to be kept in mind when illness is encountered.

Considerations in the choice of the potency.

1. the susceptibility of the patient
2. the seat of the disease (mind, emotion, physical)
3. the nature and intensity of the disease
4. the stage and duration of the disease
5. the previous treatments
6. the age of a patient
7. the constitution and temperament of a patient
8. the habits of a patient
9. the pathological conditions

When it comes to emotions, mind symptoms and chronic diseases, the high potency is effective, and lower is used for physical symptoms, like sore muscles, bruising and acute illness injuries. Medium is useful for the organs. At the end of the day a very experienced homeopath will probably know which potencies to use but in the beginning a good rule of thumb procedure is useful, so keep high potencies for chronic problems and low potencies for acute ones.

12.

How Long One Has To Wait Before Seeing An Improvement In A Very Acute Case, A Subacute Case, And A Chronic Case.

꼬

Very acute case: seconds to minutes.

Subacute case: days or several days or longer.

Chronic case: anything from a few days to four weeks or more, though Pacaud says three months.

However, there are various factors which influence changes in the above times. The patient's constitution may differ from the average, and since each patient is a unique individual, each constitution will react differently, with different power and over different time spans.

Organic or structural change within the organism may stop remedies from working altogether, or slow them down considerably, or cause them to work only partly. Sometimes these changes can be irreversible. In the case of serious damage e.g. damage to bones and joints in chronic arthritis, there may be minimum or slight improvement only, or none at all.

High potencies may cause slow improvement, on the physical side, as they work on the mentals/emotionals, and low potencies may cause quick improvement on surface ailments. The potency used will affect the time taken for an improvement. Where there is organic damage the best results are likely to be achieved with low potencies. Since these can be repeated frequently, they can be taken regularly for days, weeks or months even, until improvement occurs, when they should be stopped. They can be started again when the symptoms re-emerge.

A strong Vital Force, when jolted into action by a remedy, may immediately start working, and the patient will first feel good, and then the symptoms will start to disappear. A weak Vital Force with weakened vitality, will take longer to react, and not every single patient's Vital Force will necessarily be activated, or stimulated into action at all; or may not cope with the symptoms. If the Vital Force is weak, as indicated by the general state of the patient, and an assessment of its vitality, then too high a potency may result in a long aggravation of symptoms.

If a good simillimum is chosen, then the remedy may work rapidly, since so many of the patient's symptoms will match the remedy symptoms. However, the poorer the match, or the fewer the number of matching symptoms, the less effective the remedy may be, or the slower an improvement may be. The remedy may work on part of the illness, or only partly on symptoms, or not at all, or more slowly than a good match. An inappropriate, non-matching remedy will have no effect at all, so there could be a fruitless wait for improvement.

When there are miasms present, they may obstruct the remedy action completely, or partly, causing different time-spans of improvement. Sometimes they may cause each dose to work to lesser effect, or perhaps more slowly, until finally the remedy does not work at all, and there could be a wait forever to see any improvement.

There are certain guidelines available for us to see how long it will take for a remedy to act. Improvement may be seen, but there are other factors to consider as well. For instance, how long should one wait to see whether there will be an improvement, especially in chronic cases? Then there is the question of whether the homeopath has correctly distinguished between acute, subacute and chronic conditions, and whether the appropriate remedy has been selected in correct potency, and whether one remedy or more has been prescribed, which could change the picture. An aggravation can sometimes be an improvement and needs to be recognised as such. Similarly, a change in one symptom (or two perhaps) may be seen as an improvement but not be one.

This question refers to improvement, but sometimes there is change which can be dangerous and require an antidote. When the remedy has been suppressive, causing symptoms to move from outer to inner places, from extremities to inner organs, or upwards (opposite to Hering's Law of Cure), then this is not an improvement.

13.
Duration Of Expected Action And Repeat Dosage.

In homeopathy, there is a school of thought which suggests the homeopath take some time and effort, in order to select the correct simillimum. After the similimum is administered, everyone should wait patiently (the patient should have been appraised of the mode of operation of a homeopathic remedy), and in due course the Vital Force should respond appropriately and the symptoms, after a possible aggravation, should diminish or disappear. Although there are different durations of expected action, each case is individual, and a close watch should be kept to see if and when the action begins, and how long it endures for. Once a remedy has had its effect, even if it is still within the expected duration of time, and the effect has worn off or run its course and is no more, then the remedy can be repeated if the symptoms remain the same. If they have changed (symptoms from the outer ring of the onion model have been removed and new ones exposed underneath), then another remedy, or a different potency might be indicated.

In the case of no action from the remedy, one might consider that an inappropriate remedy has been prescribed, or a wrong potency, or perhaps a miasm is stopping any action. However, if you take Arsenicum album as an example, there is an expected action of between sixty and ninety days, leaving a full thirty days of uncertainty and a margin on either side for individual differences, stronger Vital Force etc. If a remedy has had its effect and this has not been recorded or observed, then the patient might wait for ninety days or more wondering if the remedy is going to cure him, when in fact a repeat dose may have been called for.

If a remedy is working, a repeat dose may stop the action, or slow it. If the remedy does not work within the expected time, it could be the wrong potency or the wrong remedy. A new remedy, or a different potency might be required, or increased frequency of doses. Alternatively, the patient's constitution may be different to usual animals and this may change the time spans of the remedies.

So it seems that although a remedy's expected action of duration should be understood and borne in mind, by both the patient and the homeopath, it should not be strictly adhered to, but rather the action of the first dose should be monitored and used as the guide for whether a repeat dose is necessary, within the expected duration time of that remedy.

Fundamentally, after a homeopathic dose, no new one should be administered until the effect of the first one has ceased. Patients may improve after the first dose, and need doses less and less frequently. Alternatively there may be improvement after each dose, and doses may need to be brought closer to each other until cure is effected. A greater potency may be the answer in that case. One can "plus" (dissolve tablets in water and have spoonfuls at perhaps hourly intervals if the response is good but short-lived). One can agitate the water to possibly increase or maintain effectiveness. If the remedy stops working the remedy should be reviewed and perhaps a new one tried. On rare occasions the remedy could have died in the container and the patient and homeopath could wait forever.

Vigorous illness responds to remedies vigorously. Slow or sluggish illnesses take longer to respond. Fast ones may need treatment several times an hour while they are acute, and symptoms may also change. Usually the more severe the illness, the simpler the diagnosis is. Incorrect remedies will not harm people. Slow illnesses may be treated once every day. "Average" illnesses may need treatment three to eight times a day, diminishing in number. Colds etc can be treated three times a day. When one is unsure and cannot find a guideline, it might be worth simply guessing, so as to get the treatment into action. It is better to try something, as it cannot harm the patient, than to do nothing because of being unsure. The remedy must be stopped when the patient is cured.

As can be seen above, the expected duration of the effect of the remedy may not always be taken into account, especially in acute cases, and dosage may be dependent upon the individual's actual reaction to the remedy.

14.
The Most Important Precaution In Assessing A Case.

ༀ

The most important precaution in assessing a case, as opposed to taking a case, is to ensure that no harm will be done, and that there will be no delay in the patient seeking orthodox medical aid if necessary.

The assessment includes weighting and evaluating all symptoms, and if certain criteria are present, then it is safer to refer a patient to an orthodox veterinarian, as the illness may be beyond the scope of homeopathy.

Here are some guidelines for when a homeopath should, in the interests of his patient's safety and good health, and his own interests as a bona fide homeopath, seek allopathic aid.

ༀ

1.Unexplained bleeding from anywhere.

2.Breathing is too fast and too shallow and cannot slow down.

3.Any laboured breathing, or difficulties in getting breath.

4.Severe chest pain.

5.Convulsions.

6.Delirium.

7.Temperature far too high and patient delirious. Pulse racing.

8.High fever that has persisted longer than 24 hours.

9.Severe headache, especially if accompanied by any other symptoms.

10.Unusual mental confusion.

11.Really stiff neck.

12.Grey or almost white stools.

13.Profuse urination with great thirst.

14.Dark, bloody urine (not from beetroot!)

15.Unexpected and repeated vomiting.

16.Extreme weakness.

17.Severe wheezing.

18.Yellow skin or whites of eyes.

19.Inexplicable illness or something the homeopath is quite unable to identify.

20.Unexplained weigh loss.

21.Alteration in bowel habits that is sustained and suspicious.

22.Lumps, bumps or other growths, beyond normal warts etc.

23.Emotional problems, especially if self-harm may be threatening, biting leg or gnawing feet.

24.Possible anaemia. See paleness in mouth, gums, etc.

15.
The Three Groups Of Symptoms That A Homeopath Looks For.

Symptoms are divided into three categories, the General, Physical and Mental/Emotional symptoms. In every prescribing, the homeopath should attempt to have a minimum of one symptom from each group, although this is very limited, and several from each group would be preferable, if the most appropriate remedy is to be selected. It may be that the physical symptoms are presented first, as the matter about which the patient has consulted the homeopath, who must then proceed to the others. The mental/emotional symptoms should carry the most weight in remedy selection, and are the most important for the simillimum, if the homeopath can find them.

Physicals involve the real physical matters, such as what the complaint is e.g. a sore knee, or an earache. Its history and cause should be investigated. Related symptoms should be viewed, such as what makes it worse or better and what affects it. A precise description of it should be collected. Other physical symptoms should be investigated, such as head, eyes, ears, mouth, stomach, abdomen, back, limbs and everything else. The physical group includes all matters pertaining to the physical body of the patient. Examples would be ulcers, pains, vomiting, bloat, constipation, diarrhoea, cramps, twitching, sleep patterns and nightmares. The pathology of the patient as a whole should be viewed, such as growths, moles, weakness in specific organs, frequency of catching infections and everything else. Reactions to various stimuli should be investigated to see how the patient reacts to them, for example, times of day, temperature and weather, stuffy places and fresh air, breezes, bathing, rest or motion (with details....fast, slow, gentle, vigorous). Positions should be observed, with regards to how the patient feels, such as in lying down, which side, sitting, and so forth. External stimuli like touch, blankets, pressure, movement, rubbing, massage, and noise must be viewed, together with all reactions and matters pertaining to eating and drinking, sleeping, sweating and experiencing discharges. The purpose of this part of the investigation is to see what aggravates or alleviates physical symptoms.

The generals can be started by assessing how the patient is e.g. is he hot, thirsty, cold, and does pressure or rubbing help? Is fresh air needed, and is the position comfortable or would lying down improve the overall feeling of not being ill? Does he feel restless, and is he the same at any time of day? Are there discharges and what are they like and how does he feel about releasing them? Is the symptom sided and does it appear as if only one side is affected? At what time of day does the patient feel well and fine, or the opposite? An attempted assessment of the constitutional type of the patient may be useful. There is overlap with some physical symptoms but there is a difference in that the patient is being assessed as to how he is overall, and the two must go hand in hand, to some extent. Generals do not involve specifics, such as a sore paw, or blisters on the lip, and they refer to general feeling and comfort.

Mental/emotional symptoms involve mood and behaviour. Emotional is sadness, irritability, depression, anxiety, fear. Mental is dull, confused, unable to concentrate, over-active mind, is the memory affected? Loves and hates must be uncovered, attitude to company, eating aversions or cravings, contrariness, obstinacy, impatience, loquacity, hallucinations, deliriums, concentration.

Stress symptoms are useful to collect as well, to add on to the other three categories.

Each symptom should be looked at and judged as to its importance. Is it new to the patient? Are there intensity changes? The depth of the symptom should be looked at and its level in the patient. The strength of both the symptoms and the patient should be gauged. How uniquely characteristic is the symptom of the patient's state? An assessment should be made of what effect a symptom has on the patient's ability to function as a happy, creative being. Unrelated symptoms may be simply unrelated. An acute symptom may hide chronic symptoms. A homeopath needs to look at the totality of symptoms, which means in effect, that symptoms are not islands and are not individual, but are a part of the coherent aggregate of all the symptoms. Symptoms should not be a haphazard jumble, but are grouped and viewed as functional parts of the system, as each cog and nut is part of a motor car, identifiable but part of a unity.

He should rank symptoms from "debilitating" to "irrelevant". Symptoms should be checked as to strength and persistence when evaluating any case. Irrelevant symptoms are sometimes termed "peculiar symptoms". When assessing symptoms the homeopath should consider how the patient communicates, especially body language. A points system helps to evaluate symptoms. Here is a sample one, though I do not use this one. Mental symptoms score three points. General physical symptoms (looks sick) score two points. Separate body part symptoms score one point. Peculiars can be ranked according to degree of peculiarity one to three. Rank strength and intensity of each symptom one to three. Add up the points for each grouping to reach an assessment of importance.

In seeking symptom pictures, a homeopath might follow this investigating guideline. Where is the pain, and what sort of pain is it, and how does he feel? How is it different from normal, when did it start, what was happening at the time? What makes it better, or worse? Any other changes? Has it occurred before and is he taking any medicine?

In selecting a remedy, the homeopath will find that each remedy has symptoms not in the patient's symptom picture. These should be ignored as irrelevant, provided what he seeks is there. A list of matching remedies may be constructed, consulting different charts for each symptom e.g. sore throat etc. If none fits then he can look for less detail and home in on the main matters, looking for strong symptoms rather than vague ones. If he ends up with six or more remedies, then he is looking at too many general symptoms and not at the individual. The least relevant symptoms should be crossed out. The important symptoms of the remedy can now be matched with the strongest symptoms of the case. Relevant categories of the Materia Medica should be checked out. The symptoms of the case and remedy must not clash e.g. worse for heat and better for heat, or the remedy will be ineffectual. One will never find all the symptoms of a remedy fitting all the symptoms of a disease, so should look for the nearest (similar). One should try to match the strong physical characteristics, the strong mental characteristics and the strong general characteristics. Nothing can be guaranteed, so there may need to be some experimentation with each and every patient. If one has tried four remedies without success then it might be advisable to consult another homeopath.

16.
More about the dosage.

It is most important to know that a remedy should only be taken for the minimum amount of time. Furthermore, not only should it be taken for the minimum amount of time, but it should also be taken in the smallest amount possible, to achieve the healing response. One should take one dose and then wait. The remedy should kickstart the body into healing itself. If the healing response then ceases, then one should take another dose and then wait again. Take only as much as is needed and then stop. The response will indicate that it is working and that no more dosage should be taken, until and if the response stops.

One should know, too, that in acute conditions, perhaps involving great pain or danger to life, then treatment should commence as soon as possible, and can be repeated if the symptoms do not disappear. In extreme cases a remedy may be repeated perhaps every fifteen minutes, then less and less frequently until victory is achieved over the symptom, diminishing to when necessary only. This could be days apart, or longer.

In chronic situations, low potency (maybe up to 30C depending on one's outlook and whether one is in France, the USA or Europe), remedies may be administered once or twice a day, while high potency ones (maybe 200C and higher) can be administered weekly or fortnighty and very high potency ones possibly at even greater intervals, depending on the need of the patient. In all cases treatment should be stopped when symptoms disappear, and repeated if symptoms return. This could even be years apart.

One should always be aware that an increase in the volume of the remedy taken, such as increasing the dose from one to three tablets, will not increase the effectiveness, but may in fact neutralize the good effect and/or cause aggravation and adverse reaction. Frequency is foremost a requirement, and correct frequency will ensure positive results. Watch carefully, and the symptoms will dictate the frequency of dosage.

A final note about what one should know about taking a remedy, is to be able to use one's logic in extreme cases. For instance in severe earache which has come on suddenly, a dose may be given every five minutes, but with a slowly developing 'flu twice to three times per day may be adequate. A head injury may call for a half-hourly dose. If no improvements are forthcoming then it is possible that the wrong remedy has been selected. In all cases, increase the gaps between doses as soon as progress is seen. When a strong positive reaction is seen, then stop the dosage altogether. If you continue at this point, the remedy may stop the healing process, or aggravate the symptoms.

17.
Limiting The Higher Potency Doses (More Than 30c).

Low potency remedies tend to work on tissue, and are good for acute pains like catching a tail or claw in a door. High potency remedies work on the entire creature, including the emotional and mental systems, and after three days may have a detrimental effect on patients. Patients may also start exhibiting remedy symptoms, or other morbid reactions, if they take too many high potency remedies for more than three days. Some remedies are made from deadly toxins and therefore care should be taken not to overdose.

18.
Constitutional Remedies And Categorisations.

❧

Why have healers been keen on working out constitutional types?

❧

Healers have tried to categorise patients. By taking into account physical characteristics, emotional and mental tendencies, strengths and weaknesses, and their modalities, they have tools for working out the state of balance or imbalance within the individual. This way the healer can determine appropriate healing remedies. By analysing the patient the healer can construct a picture of the patient, which in homeopathic terms is called the "constitutional picture", and which reveals the "constitutional type" of the patient. The selected remedy is chosen because it matches the temperament, character, outlook and features, historical tendencies and symptom patterns of the patient and is said to be the "constitutional remedy" for that patient.

Constitutional prescribing seeks a simplified, boxed and complete method of determining the most appropriate remedy, by trying to analyse and identify the type, then matching it to the symptoms of various remedies until, if possible, the exact match is found. This match will be the correct constitutional remedy and should cure all mistunements within the system, provided the match is comprehensive enough. It is far more comprehensive (in homeopathy) than the simple allopathic or psychological, broad spectrum type of labelling we find, such as "infection of the stomach" or "schizophrenia", which indicate a possible remedy for many different states of the same disease. Rather, numerous symptoms are exposed, and used to identify the constitutional type. Constitutional remedies are also used for maintenance of equilibrium and health, and keeping the entire system in tune. Constitutional remedies are completely personal to the patient and not generalized, in homeopathy.

It is very convenient for any healer to identify a constitutional type, so that all his further healing can be based on that model, although it may not be accurate. I have been reading about one healer who identifies all his human constitutional types by a rapid glance at their finger nails, and prescribes without delay on this basis, which to my way of thinking is over-simplified. Any similar system with animals may be flawed as well.

Numerous books have been written to assist in the discovery of constitutional types, or "bodymind homeopathic personalities". Some of the authors are P. Bailley, E.C. Whitmont, R. Sankaran, P. Chappell and many more. Some combine psychology with homeopathy, others combine pediatrics, others allopathy, and some look at up to three hundred remedies in depth.

There are literally constellations of various types of constitutional "typing" going back into history, based on various aspects of humans, such as morphology, physiology and psychology. Galen proposed his famous sanguine, melancholic, choleric and phlegmatic types. Kretshmer identified pyknics, asthenics, dysplastics, ectomorphic and endomorphic types, which have been taught at universities for decades. To me they all seem over-simplified, as humans have combinations of many things within them and all prescribing needs to be specific to each person. So far, I have not found any similar systems within the non-human kingdoms, although one cannot discount the possibility that in the future some usable "typing" may be developed by those healing birds, animals, fish and reptiles.

In homeopathy, a time came when Hahnemann found that using symptoms alone was not always sufficient to prescribe an effective remedy. He realized that the transitory symptom picture was only a part of what was required by the homeopath. This led to an evaluation of the character, the life situation, the living habits, the likes and dislikes, social and domestic relations, sex and sexual tendencies and everything else, all of which can be used to determine the constitution of the patient, which assists in the selection of the most useful remedy.

Maljonic says, look at the appearance of the patient first, then the mental and emotional aspects, followed by the physical weaknesses, then try to find the closest constitutional type. Then look at what they came about, perhaps stomach aches, and repertorise stomach ache remedies, to find several, of which one should be the constitutional remedy, which is what to prescribe.

Korean medicine traditionally identifies four basic constitutional types, Ayurvedic (simplified) three types, and other systems sometimes have more, but homeopathy has hundreds of constitutional types, being very thorough and personalised.

Once a homeopath has an overview of the patient's constitutional type, he is in a position to try to match it to the remedy which has the same profile in as many symptoms as possible. This means looking at everything about the patient, and finding, the remedy which will act upon the very core of the patient. This should activate the Vital Force in such a way that the entire system is brought back into balance and harmonised, in a manner which radiates outwards from the core, affecting first the outer ring of symptoms, and then moving inwards, casing brief flare-up and then cure of each symptom. The most recent symptom would react first, followed by the next most recent, and so on, until, all would be gone. One can compare the rings with layers like an onion has, and The Law of Cure states that the newest ones (outer) are disposed of first, followed by the others.

Of course, a deep-acting constitutional remedy, should be administered in a high potency, but locally-focussed remedies (for tissue damage, breaks etc), should be in low potencies.

In constitutional prescribing, we are using the deep acting high potency remedies to act directly upon the subtle or ethereal body to restore harmony. Because the "rings" of symptoms may stretch back from many years, or decades, this could take a long time, perhaps years. There could be brief recurrences of old illnesses, aggravations of current acute illnesses, and in certain cases more than one constitutional remedy might be indicated. Indian and Greek schools tend to favour more than one such remedy. Classical constitutional or Kentian prescribers (called Unicists in Europe), like to prescribe only one remedy at a time, so they can see which one is affecting what. They believe that ideally one remedy should encapsulate the entire patient. The Pluralists may prescribe several at a time and are sometimes termed complex prescribers, and mix remedies. I believe this approach should be made with great care as the effects may be unpredictable or unwanted. Complex remedies, such as calcarea carbonica, already consist of thousands of chemicals.

Various medicine systems identify "types" and try to link up physical characteristics, and emotional profiles, strengths and weaknesses etc to see where the internal balance is impaired. In Ayurvedic the three humours join at birth to produce seven constitutional types. In Islamic medicine, four humours combine to produce eleven constitutional types. In homeopathy we analyse the interaction of physical and mental features to find the profile of the patient and thereby identify the correct remedy. Hence we arrive at the "Arsenic types" etc. There are numerous types and numerous remedies with no strict categorisation. We match the patient profile to the remedy profile to cure the patient.

A constitutional picture may reveal a homeopathic type. Symptoms and reactions present a recognisable pattern of general physical, particular and mental/emotional symptoms e.g. a calcarea carbonica type is likely to be overweight, fair-haired, fearful and lacking in confidence, perspire on the head when asleep and crave boiled eggs. The pattern correlates with the picture of the remedy and is verified by clinical experience. Identifying a type is useful in the objective understanding of a pattern, but because of individualisation the remedy selected may differ from that of the classical type. An acute symptom may hide the details of the type, or the constitutional picture. A good homeopath should take into account the patient's type, nature and symptoms. A constitutional remedy sometimes results in an aggravation (intensification) of some symptoms before the patient starts feeling better. Cure is not measured by symptom-relief alone, but by how you feel physically emotionally and mentally. Constitutional remedies may result in anything from a very slow to a very swift cure.

What we are trying to do in constitutional prescribing, can be well demonstrated by using a Lycopodium Type, in human beings, as an example. These constitutional types tend to be thin, spare, nervous and have pains on the right hand side, appearing self-confident, but having low self-confidence, and being flatulent and feeling full after small meals. The homeopath will study the patient to determine the constitutional type, and will not merely study the disease. Constitutional types have physical characteristics, emotional profiles, strengths and weaknesses, and the homeopath can spot the internal imbalances and treat them. A type is a combination of physical and psychological factors, and the way they interact together and with their environs. The homeopath seeks a matching remedy profile. He may spot an Arsenicum, Phosphorus or Sulphur type etc and treat the constitution accordingly. In Ayurvedic or in Islamic medicine there are fixed types, but in homeopathy we acknowledge numerous combinations and seek matching remedy profiles. Thus it can be quite a complicated undertaking to successfully locate a patient's constitutional type, and more especially so if the patient cannot speak.

Constitutional types are prone to certain corresponding diseases, and constitutional remedies may cure these diseases and stop their constant recurrence, while orthodox treatment simply walls off certain manifestations (symptoms) of the disease, which will then emerge as different things. Constitutional remedies are normally administered in 30C or higher potencies perhaps monthly, although on occasion they may be given in lower potencies daily.

When a system is at ease, or in balance, it is able to detect and overcome harmful influences. When it fails to do this, it finds itself no longer at ease, but in a state of dis-ease. This can become worse and embed itself for life, and even kill the host. It can be emotional and/or physical and root causes can be multiple e.g. a fall, emotional stress, a loss of owners, an illness, or any of many others, which have resulted in the constitution no longer being able to heal itself. A constitutional remedy can restore the vigour of the Vital Force and stimulate it to cure the disease.

Homeopathic remedies have a wide range of action in certain disease states, and certain constitutions have a tendency towards certain illnesses. These do not include acute problems like accidents, psychological traumas etc. The physical symptoms of the disease can be modified by orthodox medicines to create the illusion of healing, although the chronic disease is really only being temporarily walled off and will re-emerge in different forms, only to be shot away by anti-biotics, to reappear elsewhere. The fundamental disease, mistunements or imbalances, stay in place.

By prescribing a constitutional remedy which matches the profile of the patient, one is prescribing a deep acting historical remedy which works on disease from long ago, right up the most recent, enabling the Vital Force to recognise and cure the problems.

19.
Administering The Dose In Ideal Conditions.

The homeopathic remedy should only be taken until it starts working, and then stopped, or otherwise unexpected symptoms may appear, or the remedy may be reflected by the body and not work at all. In any event the absolute minimum dose should be taken for the minimum amount of time. Homeopathic remedies in shops have recommended dosages on the labels, and this is ridiculous, in view of what I have said above. The important factor is the frequency, and not the potency of the dosage, and doses must be stopped when improvement is seen.

For animals which may be allergic to lactose, it is advisable to select other forms of tablet or liquid form of the remedy. However, pills are probably preferable to powders, granules and liquids, easy to store and take without having to sterilize droppers etc.

Tablets should be handled as little as possible, and then flicked into the mouth under the tongue or into the cheek. Those which are dropped or roll away somewhere should not be put back into the bottle but should be thrown away, as they may be contaminated with undesirable substances, or may have had their medicine rubbed off their surface. A patient may touch his own tablets, although not recommended, but other patients should not touch anyone else's remedy. One's own bugs may be acceptable to one's own system but other patient's may not be.

Tablets should be dissolved under the tongue so they can be absorbed into the system without being mixed up with too much food, other toxic substances, or stomach acids, which might make them less effective. In the case of very hard tablets, it is acceptable to chew them a little first before dissolving them under the tongue.

One tablet or dose is sufficient and gives the same benefit as two or more, no matter how big the patient is. If you struggle to get the patient to take the dose, then dissolve it in the patient's water, or at worst crush a few and put them in a little food, but food may contaminate their efficacy. In a poultry shed, for instance, it is best to dissolve a few tablets in the water.

If a patient spits out the tablets, they can be dissolved in a little spring water, stirred vigorously, and given in sips from time to time, with vigorous stirring to re-potentise the remedy fully each time. An unconscious patient can have this rubbed onto the lips, for the remedy to work.

Storage of remedies must be in cool dark areas (e.g. a drawer or cupboard), free of any strong smells or volatile substances which might inactivate them. They must be distanced from mobile phones, radiation of any sort (microwaves), direct sunlight and moisture which could damage or inactivate their efficiency. Inimical (hostile) to homeopathic remedies, may be household cleaners, perfumed cosmetics and toiletries and mints. Certain aromatherapy oils such as peppermint, camphor, eucalyptus, rosemary, thyme and lavender, may antidote or neutralise the remedies.

Beginners are advised to use low potencies e.g. 6X or 6C as these are surface action potencies which will not affect the mentals/emotionals, and they tend to act quickly to relieve acute symptoms like pain from a wound, and they stay in the system for only a short time. They are readily available in shops. Newly qualified homeopaths may use 12C or 30C until they become familiar with their actions, before possibly moving on to 200C etc. Bach remedies come in very high potencies. Higher potencies work on the mental/emotional side of the patient, and need to be understood before being used too quickly.

In very acute cases, like severe sore throats or injuries, the remedy can be taken at frequent intervals, perhaps even as close as ten or fifteen minutes apart, up to a maximum of ten, and then should be spaced out, but stopped if there is any appreciable improvement. In antibiotics, for instance, one needs to complete a course of doses, but in homeopathy one needs to stop the dose when there is any marked improvement. It can be restarted if symptoms re-appear. When patients are severely distressed it may be good to give a remedy dose every five minutes initially. Head injuries may need half-hourly doses, but 'flu may need four-hourly doses. When six to ten doses have been given and there is no improvement, then perhaps the remedy is not the correct one.

In less acute cases, with less pain, or like bronchitis, the remedy can be given two to three times a day until improvement is marked, and then stopped until symptoms re-occur. Or alternatively two tablets can be given three times a day to try to obtain quicker or more effective results.

Where there is structural damage, in the form of tissue or irreversible mechanical change, then low potencies are indicated, as in severely arthritic joints.

In chronic cases where there is no organic damage the

30C potency may be used for three days, at two tablets three times a day, but then should be discontinued so as not to produce undesirable symptoms. High potencies should be restricted to functional and emotional problems.

If new symptoms appear then stop the remedy and re-asses the case. Perhaps a "proving" is in action, or perhaps the remedy has resulted in unwanted reactions. Sometimes when a symptom has been dealt with, a new one surfaces, which needs a new remedy, or perhaps the "new" symptom is a recurrence of old ones as the Law of Cure runs its course.

An aggravation of symptoms indicates that the remedy is working, and provided it goes away, should be welcomed as an indication of successful treatment.

In homeopathy, there is a school of thought which suggests the homeopath take some time and effort, in order to select the correct simillimum. After the simillimum is administered, everyone should wait patiently (the patient's keeper should have been appraised of the mode of operation of a homeopathic remedy), and in due course the Vital Force should respond appropriately and the symptoms, after a possible aggravation, should diminish or disappear. Although there are different durations of expected action, each case is individual, and a close watch should be kept to see if and when the action begins, and how long it endures for. Once a remedy has had its effect, even if it is still within the expected duration of time, and the effect has worn off or run its course and is no more, then the remedy can be repeated if the symptoms remain the same. If they have changed (symptoms from the outer ring of the onion model have been removed and new ones exposed underneath), then another remedy, or a different potency might be indicated.

In the case of no action from the remedy, one might consider that an inappropriate remedy has been prescribed, or a wrong potency, or perhaps a miasm is stopping any action. However, if you take Arsenicum album as an example, there is an expected action of between sixty and ninety days, leaving a full thirty days of uncertainty and a margin on either side for individual differences or a stronger Vital Force. If a remedy has had its effect and this has not been recorded or observed, then the patient might wait for ninety days or more, with no cure, when in fact a repeat dose may have been called for.

If a remedy is working, a repeat dose may stop the action, or slow it. If the remedy does not work within the expected time, it could be the wrong potency or the wrong remedy. A new remedy, or a different potency might be required, or increased frequency of doses. Alternatively, the patient's constitution may be different to usual animals and this may change the time spans of the remedies.

So it seems that although a remedy's expected action of duration should be understood and borne in mind, by both the patient and the homeopath, it should not be strictly adhered to, but rather the action of the first dose should be monitored and used as the guide for whether a repeat dose is necessary, within the expected duration time of that remedy.

Fundamentally, after a homeopathic dose, no new one should be administered until the effect of the first one has ceased. Patients may improve after the first dose, and need doses less and less frequently. Alternatively there may be improvement after each dose, and doses may need to be brought closer to each other until cure is effected. A greater potency may be the answer in that case. One can "plus" (dissolve tablets in water and have spoonfuls at perhaps hourly intervals if the response is good but short-lived). One can agitate the water to possibly increase or maintain effectiveness. If the remedy stops working the remedy should be reviewed and perhaps a new one tried. On rare occasions the remedy could have died in the container and the patient and homeopath could wait forever.

Vigorous illness responds to remedies vigorously. Slow or sluggish illnesses take longer to respond. Fast ones may need treatment several times an hour while they are acute, and symptoms may also change. Usually the more severe the illness the simpler the diagnosis is. Incorrect remedies will not harm people. Slow illnesses may be treated once every day. "Average" illnesses may need treatment three to eight times a day, diminishing in number. Chills can be treated three times a day. When one is unsure and cannot find a guideline, it might be worth simply guessing, so as to get the treatment into action. It is better to try something, as it cannot harm the patient, than to do nothing because of being unsure. The remedy must be stopped when the patient is cured.

As can be seen above, the expected duration of the effect of the remedy may not always be taken into account, especially in acute cases, and dosage may be dependent upon the individual's actual reaction to the remedy.

20.

The Law Of Cure In Action.

Dr Constantine Hering formulated one of the underlying principles of homeopathy. This was The Law of Cure, which notes that during homeopathic treatment, improvement of symptoms takes place in a certain order. It begins from above and moves downwards, starting within and moving outwards, going from the major to the lesser organs and from the most recent to the earliest symptoms. The process of homeopathic treatment, as Hahnemann stated, should remove the entire cause of the symptoms, and not merely suppress the symptoms.

One might consider the sequential cause approach in this matter, and treat all identified causes in the reverse of their chronological order, because that is the direction in which the Vital Force is trying to go in its efforts to heal. To consider the course of things is to consider time, and homeopathy looks at the history of the patient to determine the direction of the cure. Usually the medical history is used to understand the symptom picture and select a remedy based on symptoms, and to identify blockages to cure. However, the sequential approach treats the medical history as the very map of the disease state, and the guide to the correct remedy.

The Law of Cure was based on a lifetime's observation of the processes involved when sick patients became cured.

Constantine Hering was a careful observer throughout his many years of practice and noted the order of the processes. They are expounded upon in a little more detail below.

As someone is cured, symptoms move from the innermost organs of the body (most vital to life) to the outer organs. Cure therefore moves from within to without. An example would be how someone with serious, life-threatening heart disease, can experience bowel problems during the process of cure.

Similarly, cure takes place from above to below, and symptoms fall away from the body, starting in the head, and clearing downwards, with hands or feet (or both) being affected last with skin eruptions.

Symptoms that have been suppressed in the past often resurface during the process of cure and usually do so in the reverse order of their original appearance. An example would be an animal, with heart disease, which had been successfully treated with orthodox medicines for a stomach ulcer, before the heart condition, and the appearance of stomach conditions would be welcomed as a sign that the old suppressed symptoms were being cleared out. The symptoms would be milder than the original illness. These laws apply to the treatment of chronic complaints but occasionally also to acute prescribing, so if an old symptom surfaces after a good prescribing, one should wait to see if it clears of its own accord. If it does, the remedy is still working and one should wait longer.

Suppression of a disease from the outside usually leads to a more deep-seated illness resurfacing. For example, children whose eczema has been "successfully" treated with steroids may suffer from asthma at a later date. These two events are seen by orthodox medicine as having only a casual connection, whereas the homeopath believes the suppression of the exzema has caused the asthma. Successful homeopathic treatment involves the eczema reappearing at some point. It is also possible to suppress symptoms with doses of homeopathic medicine aimed at single symptoms only, and not taking the whole person into account.

Homeopaths use the Law of Cure to monitor treatment and to see whether the cure is going in the right direction. As far as acute or home prescribing is concerned, occasionally a well-selected constitutional remedy will push to the surface old symptoms, that may have been forgotten. They will clear of their own accord and while they are active another remedy should not be prescribed as they might then go back in again.

It may be that any localised alteration of the state of the patient, even as small as an abscess or ulcer, is an indication that the general state is in a disturbed order. Localised imbalances can therefore be seen as barometers of what is happening inside the person, and only appear after the centre of the being has been disturbed, via the emotions, mentals and later physicals, in the order of the Law of Cure. Every acute malady begins with general disturbance, changes of temper, character, sleep, then appetite, followed by localised disturbances in the body. Cure takes place in the same way, along the same pathways, in the same order. Palliation (suppression of symptoms) for the patient's comfort or vanity, will not cure the disturbance or fundamental cause within the patient. Surface maladies are merely the external manifestations of the inner imbalance, and need to be seen as pointers to correct remedies. A good remedy will first modify the inner problems, leading to a feeling of being better, and then will follow the pattern of the Law of Cure until at the end of the process the surface symptoms vanish. The inside needs to be put in order before the exterior symptoms are approached. The Law of Cure is the homeopath's compass and rudder in his struggle to treat the fundamental disease.

21.
Modalities.

Modalities are the factors which aggravate or improve symptoms, feelings or conditions. They assist the homeopath in selecting a remedy, far quicker, by eliminating many wrong ones, and by pointing to correct ones.

There are so many homeopathic remedies for each disorder, that simply looking for "PAIN" will not find the most closely matching remedy for the specific pain. The fact that the ailment hurts is not sufficient to tell the homeopath which remedy to use. But the modalities of the pain – the kind of pain it is, where the pain is, and when it hurts most – will help enormously. These are some of the factors one needs to address. For example: if the pain pulsates and burns in the leg, in addition to having certain modalities such as worse on the left side, and in the evening, and better from cold applications, then you will be able to find the most curative remedy for the leg pain.

Modalities are always very important factors in choosing the most closely matching homeopathic remedy, to the totality of the simillimum. They can be the deciding factors between several remedies which may be strongly indicated. Modalities are the modifying influences and circumstances which either ameliorate (influences which make the symptoms of a condition feel better), or aggravate (influences which make the symptoms of a condition feel worse). Modalities include many factors and stimuli as perceived by the patient. Modalities may have to do with temperature, weather, climate, movement, activity, time, right and left side, sensations, physical contact, foods, drinks. They are the sensory manner and mode of how the symptoms are felt by the individual, and they are a most important criterion in choosing the right remedy.

Committing modalities to memory can aid the homeopath in prescribing remedies, although he must be sure of his facts.

There are innumerable modalities, but some frequently found ones are time of day, movement and position, and draughts. Environments are also modalities, making a patient feel better or worse, such as being at the seaside, in sunshine or shade, outside or inside, wet or dry, cold or warm, in different seasons, in warmth or cold, closed in or exposed, covered or uncovered, swaddled, standing or sitting, crouching or being in a fetal position. Rhythms should also be considered, such as repetitions, seasonal changes, at noon, and so forth.

Modalities are circumstances and conditions which affect or modify a particular symptom or state of a patient as a whole. They are aggravations or ameliorations of particular complaints or the state of the patient as a whole, with regard to various factors. Boericke alone lists circa two hundred and fifty modalities in his Materia Medica.

Modalities are extremely valuable to the prescribing homeopath, and rank second in importance only to the mental/emotional symptoms. Their value lies in helping to distinguish whether a remedy will work or not. For instance, one cannot expect success from a remedy which is better for heat, when the patient symptom picture is worse for heat. Modalities help to eliminate incorrect remedies quickly and help in selecting the simillimum.

22.
Something To Always Bear In Mind.

The single most important point in homeopathy.

The most important point is to match the patient's symptom profile with the appropriate remedy profile. This has been termed "The Law of Similars". It does not mean that you have to have all the symptoms in order to justify a given remedy, but the overall symptom picture should match the overall remedy profile in as many aspects as possible. The closer the match of the overall templates, the more successful you are likely to be with the remedy. Each complaint may be able to be treated with any of a group of remedies, so various guidelines are available to help select the most appropriate remedy. These include, among others discussed below, the patient's mental symptoms, mood symptoms, the acuteness of each symptom, time and space factors relative to the symptoms, aggravating and ameliorating factors, internal and external, like day or night, hot or cold, or anything affecting the symptoms, the rapidity of the onset, which side is affected, how the patient differs from his "normal" self etc, to sum up the entire picture to use for selecting the best remedy.

The "Law of Similars" seeks to find the "simillimum" or

perfect remedy for the patient at any particular time. The more complete the match of the simillimum and patient symptoms are, the more likely the remedy is to stimulate the life-force to cure the illness. It is for this reason that matters such as temperament, response to illness, actual description of each symptom (e.g. stinging, burning, stabbing pain), cravings and aversions, likes and dislikes, preferences, reactions to any aspect of the environment, and anything unusual and peculiar, are all investigated in the homeopath's construction of the most complete patient symptom picture. Orthodox medicine does not generally seek this complete picture of the patient, but focuses on each symptom in isolation. Orthodox medicine may therefore prescribe many remedies for the same ailment that homeopathic remedies can cure with one remedy. Homeopathy aims at the overall picture and orthodox medicine at each aspect as if it is unrelated to the others.

This basic principle dates back far into history, and was recognised by the Greek philosopher Hippocrates. Its Latin name is "similia similibus curentur" (like cures like), and relates to the patient's ability to cure himself when his life-force is stimulated. Only in the Eighteenth Century was it really developed in Europe. Hahnemann, the German physician, tested and developed the principle, going into fine details with the drug and symptom pictures, and naming the principle of healing, "homeopathy", based on the Greek words "homoeo" (similar) and "pathos" (suffering). He also found that with extreme dilution, he could avoid the ill-effects of drugs, and could also increase their effectiveness by potentising them.

Possibly, this point is the most important point in homeopathy, because it diverged from the standard idea that in order to cure a symptom, an antidote was administered, while in homeopathy, a substance is introduced which will bring about the same symptom in a healthy person. It constituted a move from curing with opposites to curing with similars.

23.
Best Process Of Repertorisation (Remedy Selection).

ৡৡ

In the process of repertorising, it is preferable to consider all symptoms as displayed by the patient, so as to assess the patient's own unique way of interacting with the world. Each patient is absolutely individual and unique, and cannot be "grouped" into a remedy as is done with allopathic medicine, e.g. sore throat – antibiotic. Rather, the entirety of the symptoms is viewed, and because they are not all of equal significance in remedy selection, they are generally grouped by type, and homeopaths consider the groups in repertorising each case. Of course there can only be groups when there are enough symptoms available to the homeopath, and a single-symptom repertorisation, for instance, is not concerned with groups.

The more groups that are represented in the repertorisation, and the greater the number of symptoms for each group, the stronger the possibility will be that the selected remedy will be fully beneficial.

A good manner of repertorising is simply to select each symptom, and to see in the repertory which remedies have that symptom. When all the symptoms have been thus investigated, hopefully a single remedy will be very clearly indicated. If more than one remedy is indicated, then the symptoms may be weighted according to their grouping, and the remedy with the highest score will be the most appropriate remedy. Symptoms are not all of equal value in remedy selection, and perhaps Dr Edward Bach was the most outspoken and innovative in investigating the symptom order of importance. He found that provided the mood of the patient was correct, the cure would follow, for a host of reasons....the Vital Force would become activated (in itself usually leading to cure), the patient would "decide" to get well, and correct processes would be followed, eating properly, resting, and all else necessary to get well. Therefore he invented the Flower Remedies which work only on moods to cure illness. Other prominent homeopaths and physicians have also perceived the value of the emotions, above the physical symptoms.

As a result of these insights, the symptoms **grouped under mental/emotional** should always be weighted the most heavily, or carry the highest score of all symptoms. They are the most important in the healing process, and influence the Vital Force to the greatest extent. Sometimes they are grouped as "mind" or "mind and emotions". What goes on in the head, is seen as being able to influence what goes on in the body. Personally, I have found Dr Bach's Flower Remedy symptom pictures, and the pictures of the patient after the cure, to be quite stunning in their value and insight. Attitude is so very important, and if this is right, then healing can frequently take place. So the first recorded symptoms in gradation of importance are always the mental/emotionals, except of course in acute or very acute cases, like poisoning, injury or sudden trauma, when the physical can take precedence. Also it is of importance that the homeopath distinguishes between significant and irrelevant symptoms, as irrelevant symptoms can waste time and cause inappropriate remedies to be selected. Symptoms should also be those which are not normal to the patient, although some may be so well-established that the patient's keeper does not see them as symptoms, but as normal things to live with. An example of emotional symptoms would be depression, and of mental symptoms, would be memory.

The next group of symptoms to be considered, in gradation of importance, is the group of **modalities**. Sometimes appearing in two groups called "environment" and "food and drink", these symptoms usually are preceded by the words "better for" or "worse for", or sometimes "alleviated by" or "aggravated by", and they occupy a slightly lower position of importance than mental/emotionals. They are extremely useful in selecting remedies, or in differentiating between remedies when more than one is indicated in the repertory. Typical examples would be, "Worse for hot drinks" or, "Better for fresh air". These are the factors which aggravate or improve symptoms, feelings or conditions. It is very important to master these and to look for them when assessing a case, otherwise a completely inappropriate remedy might be chosen. For example, giving Bryonia to someone who is made worse by lying still, or improved by moving around, instead of Rhus tox (see Bryonia vs Rhus tox). Modalities include addictions and aversions, or likes and dislikes, or cravings and aversions.

Finally, the lowest ranking group of symptoms would be the **physical symptoms**, paradoxically most probably what the patient was brought in about in the first instance. An animal owner might very well demand a quick palliative for his animal, such as a "homeopathic aspirin" (Mag phos) for its pain. However, the pain might appear to the homeopath, to be a far more serious symptom than the patient's owner thinks it is. The owner might think an ache is only an ache but the homeopath might see it quite differently after investigating its details, duration, modalities and history, and feel a vet should be consulted at once, or that a deep fundamental disease is responsible for it. This would involve investigating all the other symptoms which the owner might see as irrelevant, even after the truth of homeopathic remedies has been explained to him. The history of the ancestors might even become relevant, perhaps if a miasm is identified. For the sake of the owner's peace of mind, or preconceptions, the physical symptoms might have to be laboured at the cost of the mentals or modalities, although once repertorisation is in motion, the mentals/emotionals would come first, followed by the modalities, and then the physicals. However, it needs to be borne in mind that a quick-acting low-potency remedy might need to be prescribed first, to alleviate physical symptoms, before the real matter of the fundamental cause is dealt with.

Physical symptoms are many and varied, ranging from history of disease, to appearance, to body condition, to gait. Some may be visible but some may be hidden from the homeopath.

24.
The Overlap Of Remedies, Using Arnica As An Example.

There are first class, quick acting remedies for numerous first response cases. In order to convince a family of the effectiveness of homeopathic remedies, I would guess that the single remedy to convince them would need to have certain specific attributes. These attributes would need to be that the remedy is quick acting, as one with a long, protracted time of action might not be convincing. It should also keep on working and not be transitory. It should be a remedy for regular normal occurrences, and not one for the once-in-ten-years type of requirement. In fact the more often it might be used, and the stronger and quicker its action, the more likely it is to be a convincing remedy. The effect should preferably also be a rapid physical one, as other emotional, or slow responses, might be pooh-poohed as not being the action of the remedy.

The remedy should not be a male or female one. It needs to be suitable as well, for all ages, from pups/calves to the elderly. I think it should not be a "sided" remedy as this would eliminate illnesses of the other side, or ones not sided.

Many remedies act strongly on the mental/emotional aspects of a patient, and although this is good, I think that perhaps this particular remedy ought to be strongly physical, as the physicals impress people quickly and are well associated with medicines, and not tainted with shame about treatments, generally. It will be all the better, in my view, if animals can also be treated with this one selected special remedy, which should persuade any family to appreciate homeopathy.

According to a number of websites and also advertisements I have found, Arnica is the best-selling remedy in the entire world, in all its presentations, pills, creams, powders, ointments, drops, etc. (North Island Weekender ezine and others). However, it is the thirty-ninth most popular online purchase (www.abchomeopathy.com). Sulphur, followed by Lycopodium, then Gelsemium, are the most popular online purchases (www.island.net). There have been some quite serious attempts by international companies and groups to discredit Arnica, and to indicate that its does not work, but if you read the test methodology it is not very convincing. The point is that if people go to such lengths, then it perhaps indicates that it is considered a threat to orthodox doctors.

It would certainly be the first choice of my own extended family, if they were to choose only one remedy for the animals, (and themselves). It can be used for numerous ailments, within reason, as will be shown. The first choice of form would be pillules or tablets or pills or powders.

Arnica is the most commonly used homeopathic remedy in the world and once one has tried it for the treatment of injuries one might consider it a miracle remedy, and gain great faith in homeopathic remedies. (Dr Ingrid Pincott). Its success is almost guaranteed and it should be in everyone's purse or glovebox. Arnica, or Monk's Hood, can be seen flowering at high altitude, and is traditionally smeared on aching muscles by hikers in high places. The dried leaves have been smoked as a kind of tobacco in various parts of the world, and its flowers, if inhaled when freshly crushed, cause sneezing and hence its name of "sneezewort". It is much more effective in homeopathic form. It is highly recommended for any kind of trauma, whether accidental or intentional (surgery). It will reduce swelling dramatically as well as relieve pain and bruising. Surgeons wonder why Arnica–taking patients did not develop the usual bruising, and require pain-relieving medication. The best success in Arnica is in immediate use in quite high potencies, 30C and above, although it works in lower potencies too, but then needs to be taken much more frequently in higher doses. Arnica can be combined with any drug with no side-effects at all. Newborns and mothers can take Arnica to reduce the trauma of childbirth. After a sports injury it is best to take it until the injury is well on the way to healing.

This remedy can be applied in cream form to injuries that have not broken the skin, as Arnica will irritate an open wound or cut. The cream, also known as Traumeel cream, is rubbed into sore joints and muscles to relieve discomfort. Old fisherman can rub it into their hands every day to keep them limber and less sore.

With broken bones it is often felt that nothing more can be done after splinting and pain management. However there are basic nutrients and homeopathic remedies that can reduce the pain as well as speed up the healing of the bone. Initially one should use Arnica to reduce pain and swelling, before using Symphytum to aid healing of the bone and if there is deep bone pain, then Eupatorium may be used.

Arnica is excellent for rapid recovery during times of heavy training, and for the quick recovery from injuries.

Head injuries may result in residual symptoms for days

or even weeks or months, and Arnica can help greatly for this problem. Any injury to the nervous system, such as catching a tail in a car door, will benefit from Arnica, which can also be used in conjunction with various other homeopathic remedies. It is very good for relieving pain after dental work has damaged nerve-ends. Arnica will speed up healing and reduce edema and bruising after any sort of procedure where the body has been cut or traumatised.

Arnica is a highly recommended remedy for pets, especially good for bruises, and emotional or physical trauma. It is good for muscles, aches and sprains, strains and injuries, as well as injuries of the brain and spinal cord, and post-operative shock. Animals in a lot of pain, and fearful of being touched, enjoy great pain relief and calming from Arnica. Rats, dogs, budgies and horses respond well to Arnica and injured sheep naturally graze Arnica in the mountains, seeking it out themselves.

To sum up, the main uses of Arnica are as follows:

Smelly breath.

Accident injury problems, mental/emotional and/or physical.

Aches and pains, bruises, sore glands.

Any shock or associated problem of fears, memory, causes etc.

After dentistry.

Blood blisters.

Boils, small, sore.

Broken bones with swelling.

Giving birth.

Intentional injury, surgery, sport.

Whooping-cough, bloodshot eyes, chest-pain, nosebleeds.

Eye injuries.
Head injuries, lumps from knocks.
Wounds.
Joint pains, especially worse for touch.
Sprains, fetlock, lower leg joint.
Strains, over-exertion.
Some toothaches.
Insomnia after over-tiredness.
Bed feels too hard.
Cannot bear to be touched, great sensitivity to pain.
Rheumatism which cannot be touched.
Inflammation of different sorts.
Can be taken before OR after the event.
Disorientation.
Heart attacks.
High fevers.
Listlessness.
Lack of energy.
Depression.
Anticipatory anxiety if expecting a fearsome experience.
Haemorrhages, not too major.
Falls.
Hoarseness recurring.
Aversion to touch.
Too rapidly irritated.
Hypochondria.
Wanting to be left alone.
Indifference, hopelessness, poor sleep.
Fearful nightmares.
Absentmindedness, poor concentration.
Hot head, cold body.
Eczema.

Swollen elbow.
Foul smelling stools, possible faecal incontinence in sleep.

25.
The Manufacture Of Remedies. Make Your Own.

Hahnemann devised his system of "potentisation" which he used with spectacular effect in the preparation of his remedies. Since material doses of a remedy sometimes led to unwanted side-effects, he diluted them until the side-effects disappeared, and by succussing the diluted remedy he found that it became more potent. In fact with serial dilution and succussing, from groups of tens to hundreds and then to thousands, he increased the potency enormously while eliminating all side-effects. Dilution is usually conducted with forty percent alcohol (in some cases the alcohol content may be increased or change according to the beliefs of the particular manufacturer) and sixty percent double distilled water mix, in a sterilized container. After three days of soaking (although this time span is varied according to who is making the remedies, and can actually be extended in extreme cases to three weeks as with Bryonia), in the case of soluble substances, the solution is strained and becomes the "mother tincture", from which a small quantity (termed one unit) is removed and again mixed with an alcohol/water solution of ninety-nine units in size, and the mix is then vigorously shaken and jolted, a process termed "succussing", and then repeated as many times as required. In the case of 1:99 units the solution has been diluted 1C (and with each successive succussing it becomes 2C, 3C etc). When it has been repeated thirty times it becomes 30C. With each process the remedy increases in potency. Hand-made remedies are very effective, although factory-made ones are now freely available. The Korsakov machine is very useful in this regard and homeopaths are divided into three camps about the most effective way to make remedies. There are those who believe only in hand-made remedies, those who believe only in machine-made ones and those who think both are fine. It can take days to make the remedies. Excellent results are acquired with various potencies, with 30C being possibly the most popular in the UK, and was also so with Hahnemann, although Kent and the modern European homeopaths tend to use lower potencies such as 12C or 6C. In the case of insoluble in water or alcohol, substances, like Silica (Flint), the substance is ground with lactose powder in the ratio of one part flint to ninety-nine parts lactose, and then one part of the product is ground again with ninety-nine parts lactose, and then the process is repeated once more, for a third serial trituration, and then diluted and succussed in the same fashion as soluble substances. This is termed "trituration".

According to Avogadro's Law, after a 12C potency has been reached, there are no remaining molecules of the original base substance, but the medicines remain extremely effective.

Unmedicated tablets or sugar, lactose or sucrose pills are dipped into the 30C solution, which adheres to the tablet surface, and after drying, the tablets can be administered to patients requiring a 30C dose of Silica. Saturation of the pills is preferable and the process may vary a little depending on the constituency of the tablet. I have read a report about soft tablets which absorb the potentised remedy quite deeply, while other, harder tablets, are coated with the potentised remedy which stays on the surface. Pills can be purchased from various manufacturers, or can be made at home with a number of pill-making machines which are on the market, many starting with the grinding of the sugar/sucrose/lactose into fine powder before compression into a reasonably robust pillule or tablet. Tablets may be shaped differently from balls to flat to oblong ones. In my own purchases I have found that the Pinnacle tablets are a lot harder than the New Era ones, for instance.

The entire process should be kept distanced from mobile telephones, microwave ovens, direct sunlight, heat, strong odours, radiation and strong magnetic fields, and of course damp and human touch.

Medicated tablets are be stored in tinted bottles of various shapes and sizes, and kept in wooden or cardboard boxes, or leather wallets or plastic boxes, all of which keep the sun or direct light off them. They should be stored in dark, dry places like drawers. Sometimes they are kept in plastic containers with tightly sealed tops.

It is far better to treat the miasm, which will result in the disappearance of dermatological symptoms, than it is to suppress the symptoms and leave the miasm intact, which will cause it to produce more complicated and more serious problems, not necessarily skin-related either. An example of this might be that removal of warts (an external manifestation of a miasm), can result in asthma, an internal manifestation of a miasm, appearing.

It is useless to remove only one part or another of the syndrome. The remedy must be similar to all the manifesting symptoms, the background and the underlying cause. The simillimum must reflect the constitutional factors, the causation, and the totality of signs and symptoms. This is the basis of Hahnemann's miasmic doctrine.

There can also be more than one miasm present. Skin problems are only one single indicator of a possible miasm. On the same principle, Kent comments that the symptoms of asthma can never be cured unless the underlying miasm is addressed.

27.
Anti-psoric (Psoric Miasm) Remedies.

An anti-psoric remedy should be given once only, initially in high potency. Some sources say 30C and others 200C). An aggravation or healing crisis may come and go but nothing more should be given until its effect has worn off. This may take anything from days to months and in extreme cases perhaps years. The psora may have been in existence for years or even generations and cannot be cured overnight. Some examples of allopathic names for psoric symptoms are convulsions, mania, imbecility, madness, epilepsy, scoliosis, cancer, gout, haemorrhage from nose, lungs, bladder, asthma, impotence, deafness, urinary calculus, defects of the senses, and numerous types of pains. This is the tip of the iceberg only. The psora is clearly deep seated, firmly ensconced and powerful enough to kill the hosting body. The anti-psoric remedy needs time to work effectively in activating and strengthening the Vital Force sufficiently for it to recognise and deal with the miasm and all its symptoms. The Vital Force needs some time to do its job properly and restore health and balance.

There are further problems which may arise if anti-psoric remedies are given too frequently. These are that either the body may reflect the dosage, rendering it of no value, or alternatively symptoms could arise which in themselves could need further treatment. These are the inappropriate or counter-productive effects of too strong a dose. Some of the chemicals which could manifest are things such as acidity, burning, cancers, carcinomas, constipation, epilepsy, flatulence, hoarseness, itching of the skin, leprosy, burning of the spinal cord, watery discharge from nose and eyes with burning etc. There are also highs and lows, struggling with the outside world, lack of confidence, anxiety, fears, inability to cope, insecurity, but always mentally alert, with hope, to name some of them.

The psoric miasm is a disturbance in cellular homeostasis (equilibrium), making cells prone to infection and inflammation, with functional abnormalities occurring (e.g. hormone problems). The skin is usually the first to react, followed by progress into deeper, more vital organs. Bowels and lungs can be affected, resulting in inflammatory bowel disorders or bronchitis. Overproduction of cells can also result, with warts, tumours and spondylosis (spinal degeneration) occurring. Incorrect dosage could result in some of these symptoms not being addressed properly.

Miasms have mysterious and persistent progressions and only very experienced homeopaths should attempt to treat them. Hahnemann was aware of the Third Book of Moses in the Bible, (Leviticus) where the word "psora" is mentioned, referring to a proneness to disruptive diseases. Psora have been known for a long time.

Sometimes an anti-psoric remedy may work partially and many more symptoms may arise, from another previously hidden miasm or disease. These might need to be treated first before the original miasm can be treated again. Diseases and miasms can be layered, so a new assessment may need to be made after the effect of the first, single, anti-psoric remedy has been noted and observed. A series of different, possibly related remedies, may be required to remove miasmic layers. A prior knowledge of the order in which these layers have arrived, will help greatly.

This is why these remedies should be given once only, until their effect has worn off, and to see whether they are appropriate in a second or further application.

One comment which I read, was that giving too deep an acting remedy, in too large an amount, in too high a potency for the stage of the disease, results in the breaking down of the walls surrounding the bacteria, and setting it free. This related to tuberculosis and is perhaps why too much of a remedy, as mentioned above, can precipitate many of the symptoms of the remedy, or disease one is treating.

28.
Psoric And Syphilitic Miasms.

ʚAɔ

The most significant pathological (medical) difference between a psoric miasm and a syphilitic miasm.

ʚAɔ

The psoric miasm is due to some sort of suppressed itch or skin problem, while the syphilitic miasm is thought to be an inherited problem caused by syphilitic infections in past generations. The former tends to produce irritation, inflammation and hypersensitivity, with little actual tissue degeneration, while the latter tends towards granulation, degeneration and ulceration.

Physically the psora tends to make the organism toxic, the skin unhealthy, and perverts the functions of the digestive and eliminative organs. Syphilis tends to cause congenital defects, asymmetrical bony structure, deformed teeth and the classic forward-protruding lower jaw some creatures, especially human beings.

The psora is expressive and noisy, and full of self-deception. They may seem foolish and impractical. Syphilis has some madness and some genius and some irony and obsession with destruction. They can feel self-destructive (gnawing a paw for instance), and end in idiocy or insanity.

Psoric miasms result in itchy, crawling, tickling and burning pains (periodic sometimes or alternating with a congested chest), which are absent in syphilitic miasms.

Psora has scanty, irritating and itchy discharges, while syphilis has offensive, foul, putrid, smelly discharges.

Psoric skin is dry, rough, unhealthy, with little injuries becoming infected and itchy. Syphilis has brownish red or coppery coloured spots, eruptions that do not itch, and a tendency towards ulceration.

These then are the fundamental and significant pathological differences between the psoric and syphilitic miasms. However there are more, noteworthy and significant factors which highlight the differences.

Psora has restlessness and despair, dread and a tendency to forget, while syphilis has depression and self-destruction, either conscious or unconscious (see self-abuse).

Psora has a tendency to parasitic infection, like worms and fungus, which are absent in syphilis.

Syphilis has bony outgrowths and bony bumps (spine etc) which are absent in psora.

Psora is both hungry and better after rest, while syphilis is not hungry and is not better after rest.

Syphilis likes being in water, while psora dislikes it.

Syphilis has weak ligaments, with a tendency to sprains and strains, which psora does not have.

Syphilis is forgetful and loses ideas, has lymphatic and glandular problems, bloody discharges, irregular teeth and poor hygiene, of which none is common to psora.

Syphilis is better for mountains.

It is difficult for me to highlight the most significant difference between the two, as there are so many significant differences. However, I would suggest that a very significant pathological difference is the proneness to tissue degeneration in syphilis, which is absent in psora. Syphilitic conditions involve destructive processes like ulcers, many neuromuscular diseases, and ulcers, while psora produces inflammations and functional disturbances, such as dermatitis, cystitis, bronchitis, and some types of anaemia.

29.
The Bach Flower Remedies.

Bach remedies are based on personality, and so whatever the problem might be, the homeopath should select the remedy according to emotional outlook, mood, temperament and personality.

When considering Bach remedies, one focuses on the emotional and mental symptoms of the patient. They are also essential in seeking a constitutional remedy, and Bach knew that the emotional and mental symptoms should be the mainstay of one's treatment of any chronic condition. Bach's main contribution was his focus on the outlook and life of the distressed patient, rather than only the disease symptoms (physical). This was a considerable breakthrough for a physician and bacteriologist of the 1930's. He realized that disequilibrium of the mind was a prime cause of all ailments.

Using Bach as a basis, one can focus on any negative mental states which are preventing the body from healing itself. Bach found that we can classify animals (including people) into groups by the way they communicate, eat, use body language and move, and thereby display their mental states. Giving up his practice, he investigated the situation further, so paving the way for homeopaths of the future to be able to recognise and cure negative states, which prevented cure. When using Bach Flower Remedies we focus on the details of the patient's mental state, and change the state by administering the appropriate Flower Remedies. Once happiness is restored, in the form of inner harmony, the creature thinks clearly, does the appropriate things to cure itself, effects internal cure by using the Vital Force, and throws off the mood which had brought it down. If not treated soon enough, bad attitudes and moods can snowball into major states of unbearable anguish and ill-health, which sometimes include very anti-social behaviour patterns.

We know that when a system is out of balance or mistuned, a negative state creeps in, which can be associated with either personality, or be a transient mental state created by the circumstances and conditions of life. Look at home change, bereavement, disappointment, isolation, infirmity, unpleasant environments, and you find anxiety, anger, depression, impatience, unhappiness, and these alter the system's well-being and it feels ill and look older. Edward Bach knew this and treated the negative outlooks with flower remedies. Homeopaths follow suit and look for negative outlooks when considering flower remedies.

Bach identified seven basic groupings for us to consider. Each group headed the emotional states curable under that heading. He developed thirty-eight remedies to cure these negative states. Homeopaths need to focus on each heading, and then its subsections, when considering the flower remedies. It must be borne in mind that many of the emotional states may not or do not apply to all or most creatures which are not human. They are, briefly:

Fear – terror, panic, fears, shyness, of the unknown.

Uncertainty – of judgement, need others, moods, dejected, despair, fatigue, indecision.

Lack of interest – dream, escape, apathy, drifting, gloom.

Loneliness – quiet, intelligent, impatient, intolerant, self-interested.

Over-sensitive to influence and ideas – inner torture, weak, habits, hate, jealousies.

Despondency and despair – overwhelmed, shock.

Over-care for welfare of others – possessive, ruthless, leaders, overworkers.

By focussing on the above we can select a Flower Remedy. There are also remedies available for no less than six sleep disorders, including unwanted thoughts, and also a Rescue Remedy for all traumas and shocks.

When considering Bach remedies, we need to remember that good health is harmony, rhythm, positivity, constructivity and general happiness. Ill-health is negativity, unhappiness and destructive attitude. The entry of Bach, into the world of emotions in diagnosing health, started when he found that fear caused asthma in a patent. On this he developed his life work.

What Bach believed his remedies would do.

Bach believed his remedies would cure gloomy attitudes, aloofness, hatred, envy, self-despising and other negative emotional states. He believed that in turn, this would enable the patients to heal themselves, as nature intended. Bach was a very staunch Christian and believed God had made creatures to be self-healing if only the negative emotional states could be cured. Bach used extremely high potencies to work on the emotionals, including positive and negative attitudes. He believed his remedies would even cure deep resentment, and of course every other possible negative emotional state.

Looking further, Bach felt that disease was manifested in the physical body because of the resistance of the personality to the guidance of the soul. The soul (intuition) guides via instincts, desires, likes and dislikes, which are things good for that personality. These things will forever be present and often dormant until they are indulged and the soul is satiated. The world and those around, judge and condemn, and try to force creatures in directions, opposite to their soul cravings (see cages for animals and offices for humans). Disease results because of the resulting moods and emotional reactions e.g. sadness, anger, fear, anxiety, aggression and many more. The ultimate selfishness is to try to control other creatures.

The personality is destroyed and damaged by the pressure of dominant and ugly creatures, but Bach remedies strengthen the personality to allow it to overcome the obstructions of life. Disease is merely a symptom of the cause, which is disharmony.

Radiance, happiness, or whatever you wish to name it, is the harmony of the soul and the physical self. Logic is not required as feeling and emotion tell the entire story. Bach believed his remedies would help to restore this feeling when it was temporarily lost. They help creatures to overcome convention and the unnecessary trivialities of life.

Outlook, harmony and attitude all change hardships to adventures. Bach knew this and focussed on moods, perceptions, emotions and attitudes. All Bach remedies work on the mind and the body receives the "spinoff" so to speak, of health from a healthy attitude.

He believed his remedies could lead to health via love, sympathy, peace, steadfastness, gentleness, strength, understanding, tolerance, wisdom, forgiveness and courage and joy. The remedies take away the causes of disease, which are restraints, fear, restlessness, indecision, indifference, weakness, doubt, over-enthusiasm, ignorance, impatience, terror and grief. Orthodox medicine has not understood these causes, and attributes disease to the symptoms only, e.g. asthma or pain.

Health is happiness, in small things, doing things one loves, being with creatures one likes, no strain, no effort, no unattainable aims, just ourselves, no false senses of duty, and no hardship-inducing ambitions. Imagine the unhappiness of animals in circuses, or some police-schools, or the plight of performing bears. It is no wonder they die far earlier than their counterparts in happier circumstances.

The stages of healing any disease are quite clear...peace, hope, joy, certainty, wisdom and love. Bach believed the homeopath should work through these layers with his patient, using the flower remedies.

In identifying what to treat creatures for, or how to encourage keepers to identify animal problems, the Bach method might be to look for the faults one hated to see most in other creatures. There could be several in number and they might be graded and treated in order of severity, worst to least hated. A remedy, plus love and sympathy, both received and given, can cure most ills. Bach believed that good overcomes evil. Disease is merely a corrective measure, an indicator to us that something in the soul is amiss. We must heed the warning. Wrong-doing and wrong-thinking is bringing about the disease. Bach believed that coercion or possession of another human (creature) is even worse for our health than material greed and power struggle. He said coercion would result in our being afflicted with the same unhappiness and ill-health we spread, and we would reap what we sow. Thus a cruel animal-keeper might make the animal diseased because of his cruelty, but would make himself diseased at the same time.

Each of the flower remedies enjoys its own personality, and is anthropomorphised into speaking, hoping, helping etc. Bach's descriptions of each are quaint and moving, especially Centaury and Oak.

The remedies were collected and proven across the length and width of the UK, and carefully logged in maps by Bach and his followers, mainly Nora Weeks. He persevered in the face of criticism and disapproval of the established medical profession and The General Medical Council, believing his remedies would cure people. In time he developed his type of remedies which rapidly assisted cure in the various mood problems, and proved his ideas to be true and valid, in the face of conservative criticism. A great deal of criticism still exists, in the ranks of the uneducated, or those with interests in suppressing non-orthodox medicine, for one reason or another.

To really appreciate what Bach felt, or knew his remedies would achieve, it is worthwhile reading his "The Story of the Travellers", where one can find outlined the emotional problems facing certain remedies, and then see what each remedy can achieve.

Bach's greatest break with tradition was the decision to break with treating the physical body and to treat the organism purely from the mental/emotional point of view. Criticisms have been levelled against Bach, that he was over-religious, thinking he was possibly guided directly by God, and also that he was too reliant upon his inner urges which could be detrimental to people when they took precedence over common sense. Perhaps he did suffer from some delusions, but they did not stop him from developing a very efficient and useful new form of treatment for diseases.

The reason for the inclusion of so much of Bach, in this book, is that animals have very similar emotional systems to humans, and sensitive healers can sometimes log in to animal feelings, and can use Bach remedies very effectively. Rescue Remedy, in particular, works very well for animals after traumas like surgery, near escapes, abandonment, floods or fires.

30.
Bach's Rescue Remedy.

ക

Rescue Remedy, its constituents and what each component is useful for.

ക

From his thirty-eight single remedies, Dr Bach formulated a special combination remedy called "Rescue Remedy", designed to help patients cope with life's ups and downs. It contains five of the original remedies, being Impatiens, Star of Bethlehem, Cherry Plum, Rock Rose and Clematis. Its gentle action works with the system to help restore a positive mood and can be used during times of shock or trauma. It is equally good for going to the vet, doing a circus act, performing at a dog-show, or being threatened by invaders like wolves. It helps with trauma such as deaths and relationship breakdowns, acute shocks and mental or physical trauma which has lead to emotional shock. It is useful for all emergencies.

Rescue Remedy may be taken internally (pillules, tablets, powders, sprays or drops) or applied externally (cream or liquid) to stings, strains or bruises. It also alleviates mental anguish, so enabling the body to start the healing process without delay. Animals which have suffered from any shock or terror will benefit from this remedy. Some plants respond well to a few drops of the remedy. Bach selected the five elements of Rescue Remedy because he felt they combine to form an effective all-round crisis remedy, as he first demonstrated with shipwrecked sailors who recovered amazingly after being dosed with it.

The uses of each component are listed below, and then expounded upon briefly:

Impatiens: tension and stress.
Star of Bethlehem: shock.
Cherry Plum: desperation.
Rock Rose: terror.
Clematis: feeling weak, lacking nerve power.

1. Impatiens, as the name suggests, is useful for treating irritability, nervousness, impatience, frustration, rush, impetuosity, and mental tension. It encourages less haste, relaxation, tolerance, gentleness and acceptance. Patients learn to wait, become less fretful and regain their poise.

2. Star of Bethlehem is indicated wherever there is shock, distressing events, bereavement, pain and, sometimes stemming back to events of years before. It can neutralize sudden or delayed shocks and sadness, and is a welcome comforter and soother. Fright can also be treated with this remedy.

3. Cherry Plum is indicated in treating patients whose minds do not cope with life anymore. It is indicated for those with self-harming behaviours. Sometimes there can be sudden murderous and violent impulses with complete loss of control. Cherry Plum can restore calm, quiet courage, and the ability to survive and endure.

4. Rock Rose is the treatment for extreme fear, terror

and panic. It may not be rational but is very real. It may be caused from mimicking other panic-stricken creatures, near escapes, seeing catastrophes, nightmares or approaching tornadoes. The terror may prevent normal behaviour patterns such as going to sleep, for terror of nightmares. It is worth noting that Rock Rose is indicated for fear which creates terror and panic, and not simply for known fears when Mimulus would be indicated. It restores courage, strength of will and character, and the ability to care for others first.

5. Clematis is indicated for nervous weakness, lack of interest in the present, a vacant look, inattentiveness, obliviousness to surroundings, boredom, lack of concentration. There is absentmindedness, sleepiness, listlessness and withdrawal. The remedy inspires lively interest, action and realistic down to earth activity.

By combining all these positive actions of the remedies, Bach came up with a general, all-purpose Rescue Remedy for many of the problems afflicting creatures. Fortunately it works equally well on humans and animals, who have simpler, but just as important emotional systems.

31.
The Placebo Effect.

This phenomenon has been so well publicised over the past few decades that it needs no introduction here. Suffice it to say that a body receiving what it perceives to be a curative substance, will sometimes cure itself spontaneously, even if the substance is inert (a placebo).

Over the years, various closed-minded people, and bigots, have tried to discredit homeopathy, some saying it is merely a placebo effect that we see. In their ignorance and vitriol, they choose to disregard the millions of human adults, babies, birds, aquatic creatures, reptiles and animals which are healed or assisted across the world every single day. In the testing of homeopathic products, the people they are tested on are frequently unaware of what they are taking, thinking it is merely a sugar pill. Babies never know what they are taking, and neither do birds, animals, fish or other reptiles, yet they respond in the same way, to the same remedies.

Arnica, for instance, has the same effects on any creature anywhere in the world.

The author has no experience of using homeopathic remedies on plants but is aware that various people have tried them and had excellent results. Silica, for instance, can perk up a drooping plant.

Crocodiles, which suffer from similar medical problems

to humans, such as influenza, respond to conventional drugs in the same way as we do, and also benefit from homeopathic remedies. Of course there may be instances, as is the case with orthodox medicines, and many complementary therapies, where a placebo effect does cure a patient, and everyone should be grateful for this happening.

32.
Tissue Salts.

❧

Included in the huge range of homeopathic remedies, are twelve inorganic tissue salts. Bodies have a critical need for each of these to be present in the correct balance and quantity, in order for them to be free of disease and pain. Below is a list of them all, their functions, and what occurs when there is a deficiency or imbalance.

The full scope of tissue salts is far beyond the scope of this pocket guide, but any animal owner would do well to read this section carefully, and to bear it in mind. Brief details of what the salts may cure, can be found in the Materia Medica near the end of this book.

❧

Calc fluor: Glandular tumours, venous problems, prolapses, bone problems. This salt is an essential component of bone surfaces, elastic fibres and tooth enamel. When elasticity is gone, then serious problems can ensue. These include the dilation of blood vessels, tumours, piles, enlarged veins, heart enlargement, relaxed (flabby) inner organs and prolapses.

❧

Calc phos: Anaemia, bloat, bone problems, development of the body, teeth. A shortage of this salt results in bone disease, and bones remain weak and undeveloped if deprived of it in the developmental stages. It plays a major part in the digestion and absorption of nutrients. Absence or shortage of it may produce anaemia, spasms, convulsions and rotting teeth. It is essential for recovery from wasting diseases, and restores a shortage of red corpuscles. Young creatures deprived of this salt, display emaciation, suppuration of bones, and spinal weakness. Later on, fractures will not heal, rheumatism may appear, and certain glands may enlarge significantly. Faeces may be hot and disgusting, with a generally sick stomach and vomitting.

Calc sulph: Catarrh, boils, suppuration, carbuncles. A shortage results in various abscesses, and is an excellent remedy for all ailments where pus-formation is liable, or has already developed. It is good for lung diseases, with heavy, yellow pus anywhere in or on the body.

Ferr phos: Congestion, inflammation, fevers. A good remedy for early stage congestion, inflammation and fevers, since it attracts oxygen and assists oxygen transportation in the blood. It strengthens the walls of blood vessels and supplies the red colour in blood corpuscles. It is excellent for anaemia, pneumonia, inflamed rheumatism, nosebleeds, incontinence and apoplexies. Symptoms are aggravated by motion.

Kali mur: A second stage remedy for inflammatory diseases, croup, catarrh, pneumonia, swollen glands,

Eustachian deafness and diarrhoea. It is good for all inflammations and exudations, and should follow Ferr phos. Second stage symptoms involve thick, white expectorations with a white or grey covering of the tongue. There may also be skin eruptions with yellow-pus pimples, ulcers and rheumatic swellings. Car-sickness is common.

❧

Kali phos: Brain, nerves, muscles, blood vessels. Supplies the brain's nerve fluid. This salt is a good remedy for sleeplessness and nervous conditions, and any nerve degeneracy (neurasthenia). Some examples would be, no nerve power, prostration, mental exhaustion, brain-fag, forms of insanity, forms of paralysis, epilepsy, hysteria, no co-ordination of extremities and blood decomposition. Examples include haemorrhages, gangrene, carrion-smelling diarrhoea, typhoid, incontinence, itches, dizziness, breathing problems, wheezing, headaches and a dark yellow tongue. The patient cannot stand noise or physical activity.

❧

Kali sulph: Third stage of inflammatory or catarrhal condition, diarrhoea, skin diseases, rheumatism, ulcerations and flatulence. The salt carries oxygen, which is a body's primary source of fuel, so therefore it is the fountain of all vitality. It assists with yellowish, watery secretions with a slimy, yellow tongue, and is good for inflamed throats, coughs, pneumonia, skin diseases with yellow pus, diarrhoea and eye problems. It may be used for scurfy or scaly skins and various ailments, which are much worse when the patient is warm.

❧

Mag phos: Spasms, cramps, convulsions, epilepsy. This salt is a constituent of muscle, nerves, brain, bone, spine, teeth and blood corpuscles. Shortage of the salt causes spasms and convulsions, and is related to nerve cells and muscle tissue. It can help in tetanic contractions, twitches and jerks, fits, coughs, paralysis and retention of urine. It is used for pains in the head, face, teeth, stomach, heart and limbs, and has been described as the "homeopathic aspirin". Sometimes there is prostration with an extremely tympanic abdomen, with flatus. There may be dysentry. Pains may move around and are sudden and piercing. Massage and warmth may help.

Nat mur: Catarrh with watery secretions, as in skin disease, constipation, diarrhoea, hay fever, colds and influenza. This salt regulates the volume of water in each cell of the body. It is found in every single cell of the entire body, both in liquids and in solids. Distribution of water within a system, if not as it should be, can cause dryness in some places and too much wetness in others. Mucus membranes react violently to this. Dis-equilibrium may also occur in the lymphatic system, blood, spleen, liver and stomach linings. Non-optimal distribution causes headaches, stomach aches, general aches and problems with secretions like tears, mucus or water, which can be too little or too much. This remedy can help with wet mucus-froth from skin eruptions, watery blisters with crusts and various other skin problems. Constipation or very wet eyes can sometimes be treated with this salt, as can eye infections, slimy bubble-covered tongues and coryza from anywhere. Other diseases of the pharynx, bladder, chest and some glands can also be cured.

Nat phos: Intestines, diarrhoea, worms and sour-acid vomitting. This salt assists in the elimination of both excess sugar and lactic acid. The latter can be a residue of physical overstress, and leave stiffness and pain. The remedy also reduces sour acid belching, fermentation, vomitting and green, stinking diarrhoea, with colic and spasms caused by mouth acid. The tongue is wet-yellow, with yellow discharge, a sure sign indicating this remedy. The eyes may release yellow pus. The bladder function may be affected and worms may take hold in the gut. Rheumatic pains often accompany these symptoms, together with itches, skin problems, crusts and pain.

Nat sulph: Liver, nausea, diarrhoea, asthma, edemas and breathing problems. This salt eliminates all extra water from the blood and regulates bile. The tongue is dark brown-green or grey-green and stools are dark green and full of excess bile from the liver. Vomitting occurs. The remedy helps with fevers, vomitting and bilious diseases. The liver is enlarged with skin eruptions and blotches. Urine may have sediment in it and skin diseases may be visible, including edemas, warts, gout-like problems, moist, yellow scales and inflammations, worse towards the front and head of the animal.

Silica: Uterine disorders, indurations, swollen glands, carbuncles, ulceration and suppuration, foreign bodies stuck under the skin (splinters, thorns, quills). Silica is critical for all functions of the body and is only less prolific than water, in bodies. This salt acts on bones, joints, glands, skin and mucus membranes. A shortage of it results in signs of malnutrition and is excellent for undernourished patients. All ulcerations and suppurations benefit from it, as do all tendons, the periosteum and the bones. Both hardness and induration can be treated with this salt, which ripens suppurations, resulting in the escape of pus. Hard, swollen glands may ripen, and drain, lie this. Constipation may be present. The eyes may be stye-infected and epileptic fits may occur, especially with moon changes. There can be flatulence and serious lung infections, with all the symptoms much worse at night. Full moon can precipitate various symptom attacks.

33.
The Organon (Set Of Scientific Principles).

An introduction into the original thoughts of Samuel Hahnemann, the father of modern homeopathy.

The physician's duty is to cure the disease in the least harmful and shortest way possible. To do this he must treat the totality of symptoms, meaning absolutely all symptoms, emotional, mental, physical, historical, lifestyle and everything else. He should not speculate on the metaphysical, nor the nature of the disease, but should simply collect every scrap of information, so as to match the appropriate remedy to the disease, so as to cure it. Palliatives for isolated symptoms are not a part of homeopathy.

The Vital Force is life. Without it there is death. With it deranged, there is disease. The guide to the derangement, and to the cure, is the complete list of symptoms. Treating individual symptoms is a mischief.

Medicines cause an alteration of the Vital Force. They are studied by what they do. The derangement they can cause in a healthy individual, is the same disease they can cure when administered to a patient exhibiting all the facets of that derangement.

Allopathic (orthodox) medicine, is the medicine of opposites e.g. when a patient has diarrhoea, then give him medicine which stops diarrhoea. Homeopathy is the medicine of similars, which administers a remedy which will cause diarrhoea in a healthy patient. This causes the Vital Force within the patient, to cure the same disease, when administered to a patient suffering from diarrhoea.

Scientific, or attempted scientific explanations, are simply pointless. The homeopath works on facts, not speculation or metaphysical dreams.

Bodies fall ill when susceptible to disease, because of derangement. An artificially introduced disease excites the body to eliminate the same disease if it is present. Introduction of a different artificial disease will not excite the Vital Force to eliminate a disease which is present. Allopathic drugs only suppress diseases, which later become chronic problems, and these drugs in themselves can cause chronic diseases and early death.

Homeopaths who prescribe palliatives, to avoid the problem of seeking the correct remedy, and to bring the patient back for more, are the lowest form of life in the world of physicians.

Summary so far.
All diseases are groups of symptoms that can be cured by similar remedies. The physician's task is to investigate the disease, investigate the remedies, and match them as closely as possible.

Acute diseases arrive suddenly and burn our brightly and rapidly, or become chronic. Chronic diseases are long-lasting, slow developers, sometimes caused by miasms or allopathic medicines. Hahnemann identified three main miasms, the Psoric, the Syphilitic and the Sycotic, though a number of newer ones have since been added.

Casetaking requires patience and listening ability, and the encouragement of the patient to talk for as long as necessary. It may even take days, but normally a few hours can deliver up a good lot of information. The physician needs to be expert at encouraging the patient to speak about literally all matters pertaining to himself. All peculiarities need to be noticed, and especially all changes noticed by the patient. Chronic diseases have masses of information and sometimes very long histories, but acute ones may have very little.

Epidemic diseases are analysed by the totality of symptoms from a number of patients.

Once the physician (homeopath) has noted all aspects of a disease, and has administered a remedy, he can diagnose the patient for feedback, and list the symptoms which have been cured. This way he can asses the effect of the medicine.

The physician needs to be able to access complete remedy pictures. He cannot experiment with them and hope for the best. Symptoms are guides, live and dynamic, to the remedy and cure

The organism is a dynamic, vibrant, living entity, a microcosm in its own right, and fully aware of every malfunction, disease or injury anywhere in or on itself. It should be treated as an entity. The treating of individual symptoms as if they stood alone, is a nonsense.

When a chronic disease is resisting cure, the physician must look for and treat miasms. A miasm may be responsible for the patient being unable to recognise and cure his disease, which has been caused by a miasm, and is being perpetuated by a miasm.

Of course all of Hahnemann's observations related to human beings, and the reader should take note of, and use, the principles which can be applied to animals.

34.
Animal Emotions.

Whether one is using usual homeopathic remedies, or Bach Flower Remedies, the effect of the remedy will only be complete when the emotional symptoms of the patient are graded as the most important symptoms when selecting a remedy. Some people are so unspoiled and unselfish, so a part of nature and the universe, that they are in harmony with other creatures, and are able to accurately identify their emotional problems or conditions. Animals have the same emotions as we do.

For instance, I know a crocodile man who had to treat an immense female crocodile for depression and indifference/ lack of interest after she had her lower jaw bitten off by another crocodile. She recovered perfectly but had to be fed from then on, and lives on the Natal South Coast in a Crocodile Park.

I have treated dogs for social anxiety, rages and aggression. Camels, elephants and swans can suffer tremendous grief when they lose a partner or parent (young camels cry huge camel tears for days on end and elephants can grieve for months). One of our camels grieved to death after her partner was killed by an oryx. Rats can experience panic when a friend disappears or dies, and break out of their cages to go in search of them. Some snakes can be filled with revenge and lie in wait for humans who killed their partners.

Buffaloes can be filled with quiet, consuming rage and set ambushes for hunters, so as to kill them. Baboons brought up in human families can experience serious anxiety when separated from their families. Orang-utans can slip into a deep apathy when removed from their families and homes and put into cages. Bears can die twenty years earlier than normal, from heartbreak, when caged or put into circuses. Domestic pets can slip into deep depression when they feel abandoned in kennels, when their families go on holiday. The story of "Boggom" and "Voetsek", the inseparable baboon and dog, is well known in some areas. One died, and the other grieved to death. Other creatures also exhibit the same stress reactions as we do, as cruel experiments on monkeys and rats have shown. The list is endless.

A final consideration is the grief experienced by humans when their pets die. The love they have received from the pets has been real, unconditional, unrelated to how they have looked or behaved, and a source of happiness and comfort. The grief experienced is deep and genuine, and often every bit as painful as the grief experienced when a human dies. Sometimes it is so bad that people vow never to have another pet, but soon change their minds, fortunately.

35.
Chinese Medicine And Homeopathy.

☙

Chinese diagnoses, and healthcare approaches, developed well over three thousand years ago, while homeopathy developed only two hundred years ago. Yet they have a great deal in common, and perhaps we shall find that Dr Hahnemann in fact had some background knowledge of Chinese medicines. The same diseases are spoken of, both in symptom form, not named form, and both rely upon quite sophisticated observations of the patient and of the effect of remedies.

The difference in the remedies, is that in homeopathy the herbal remedies and substances are diluted and succussed in a different way to the manner in which the Chinese administer them. Nevertheless, the same remedies are frequently used.

Both systems are holistic and consider and recognise the complete interaction between all parts of the body and mind, not treating symptoms in isolation, as is the way with orthodox medicines.

Western so-called "scientific analysis", is reductionist, attempting to label and isolate each symptom on its own. Chinese medicine and homeopathy look at the interplay of the body, mind and spirit, and their connection with the entire universe, and try to restore harmony within this dynamic interaction. Any disharmony signals disease.

36.
Helpful Hints In Relating To Animals.

Many animals have a deep gentleness with their own young, as well as those of other creatures. One example of this is our own two giant razorback bushpigs, who used to come out of the bush every day for a chat and a snack or drink. They loved to share an ice-cream cone with my own babies, sitting in the sand. Not once did they ever even bump the children over, or upset them in any way at all. Another example is the hippo, who almost killed a crocodile to rescue a small antelope, and then gently held the antelope's head up, with its huge jaws, until the antelope finally died from the crocodile bites, upon which the hippo slowly lowered its head to let it lie on the ground. There are hundreds of examples of animals protecting and saving young creatures. I knew two wild baboons, which zealously guarded the lambs on a nearby farm every year, making sure no jackals, hyenas or big cats caught them. They would sometimes carry weak lambs home at night, stroking them and talking to them. In a terrible tragedy, a passerby saw this happening one evening, and thinking the baboon was eating a lamb, he shot her dead.

When you are confronted by spiders or snakes, in your house, a broom can be very useful and humane in removing them. Spiders will climb onto the broom and can be shaken off outside, while small snakes can be gently coaxed to the door.

Animals may have long memories too. My friend Roy, had a baboon which adopted him, when it was very young (we did wonder why, and teased him sometimes). It went everywhere with him, onto all his building construction sites, but finally started to become too protective, so he decided to take it to a game park. He was advised not to visit it for a year, to allow both of them to settle emotionally. When he did visit, a year later, he entered the enclosure and the baboon gave a fearsome shriek, and leaped onto him. It was bigger than a Rottweiler and had long, powerful teeth, and it hugged and groomed him for the better part of the day. However, at closing time, it was quite happy to go back to its own home and supper. Elephants, sheep and fish have also been shown to have long memories.

If you ever have to move an injured creature, perhaps a vulture, dog or serval, and fear the animal, then it is a good idea to use a heavy, thick blanket to throw over it. You should also wear heavy, leather welding gloves, and if you are careful, you will easily be able to take it to a place of care. Do be careful though. We had a vulture rip the leather seats of the Peugeot 403 to shreds, before it got out and flew away.

It is never a good idea to keep snakes in bags, as they bite people through the bags, especially when people are carrying the bags or sit on them by accident. Use large plastic rubbish bins with lids, to transport snakes. In my decades of snake-catching, there were many incidents of snakes jumping high out of containers. A medium-sized female green mamba can quite easily propel herself two metres into the air, like a spring. A skaapsteker can easily jump 1.5m into the air. Some timid, poisonous snakes, may knot themselves around a branch and refuse to move. I have seen a mamba stand up on a small section of tail, to go over a two metre high wall. It is by far the best to run away from any snake, unless you have an experienced snake-catcher with you.

37.
Confrontations With Animals.

Remember that all animals can be dangerous, and what I say may or may not work.

In any confrontation with baboons, gorillas, or any other species similar to yourself, make sure you never look one in the eye. This would be tantamount to a challenge. Immediately squat down, making yourself as small as you possibly can. Turn away from the creature and waggle your rear end at it, while picking up sticks and leaves and nibbling them. If the animal comes nearer, hold your hand out to it, palm-up, while looking at the ground. Under these circumstances it is extremely unlikely that it will harm you, although it may posture a bit. This system can occasionally work with human authority figures too, but be careful when and where you try it.

There may be an occasion when you come face to face with a large, scary animal, not too much like yourself. Maybe it will be a bear. Whatever it is, never ever look it in the eye. Never turn and run away either, as animals can run very much faster than you can, and your running could trigger them into going after you. Never be too hasty to climb trees either, unless you are certain the animal cannot climb. Bears and the big cat family can zip right up trees very quickly, to pull you down. It is safe to climb trees to escape from rhinos, buffaloes, and those sorts of animals.

Stand very still when the confrontation occurs, then move backwards very slowly, making absolutely certain you leave a path of escape open to it. Never corner any animal. Look downwards and speak in a low, soothing, gentle voice, initially, before softly singing "The Teddy-bears' Picnic". Try not to sing in a high-pitched quaver. This entire procedure may save your life, but then again, it may not.

The First Response.

✌

Introduction.

Homeopathy has helped millions and millions of people, animals, birds and aquatic creatures around the world for hundreds of years. It is a wonderful form of healing, with no side-effects or dangers involved.

Dosage is effected by popping the pillule/powder/liquid into the mouth of the patient where it is quickly absorbed. The patient may be of any sort, from a chicken to a hippopotamus, to a guinea-pig, to a dog. The remedy may be dissolved in drinking water, or in extreme cases mixed with food.

Selection of a remedy for humans involves an analysis of the patient's emotions, mental processes, modalities, cravings and aversions, sidedness, history, other factors and the presenting symptoms. We are not always able to do this in the case of animals, so frequently use only the **presenting symptom**, which may be insufficient.

This "First Response" is a **very brief field guide to symptomatology in the animal world**, insufficient for human prescribing, generally, although of possible use in emergencies. It should be supplemented, where possible, with consultation of a good Materia Medica such as Boericke, where more information for each remedy can be found, and a better choice made. **The more points that match the patient, the better the chances of cure are**.

An understanding of **dosage** is important. Stop the dosage the moment there is any improvement, and re-dose if improvement stops. In a crisis you may need to administer six doses in a day (but then stop or change remedies), but normally one remedy may do the trick, or one dose per day for few days. You need to observe the effects and make your own judgement. If improvement occurs and you continue the dose, the effect may cease permanently. Some remedies may act days later. Big or small patients need the same dose. Use your savvy.

Strength of dose? I suggest 30C but others all seem to work as well. Try the suggested remedies one at a time until one works. Some organisms do not respond to any medications, but most of them do.

Common maladies are listed in alphabetical order below. It is a good idea to have a separate note book to record all treatments and results. Fairly common remedies are suggested with as much overlap as possible so you do not need to buy too many to keep in stock. There are thousands more than are mentioned here. **Run your eye down the bold listings**, to rapidly locate the ailment, followed by a possible emergency remedy. Later a proper repertorisation should be carried out.

It is strongly recommended that you carefully read through all the notes here, and familiarize yourself with the layout, as in an emergency people fail to think clearly and may not be able to locate the most appropriate remedy. **Browse the "First Response" regularly** and become familiar with everything in it.

Bach's Flower Remedies can be most effective, and are in themselves complex and complete. They work on the body via the emotional system, and are not prescribed in this "First Response".

Names of remedies are the same the world over, which

is very useful. Shortened forms may differ e.g. Bryonia may be Br, Bry, Bryon.

❧

A.

❧

Abortion: (after)
Arnica, China.
See also: Sabina, Sec, Puls, Rhus tox.
Threatening: Trill.

❧

Abdominal distention:
Carbo veg, Puls, Kali bich.
No appetite: Cham, Lyco, Nux v.

❧

Abscess:
Hep sul, Sil, Pyro.
Stinking: Merc sol.

❧

Afterbirth:
Stays behind: Saba, Sec cor.

❧

Ageing: (see trembling)
Ambra gris, Berb vul, Vera alb.

❧

Aggression:
Bell, Nux v, Sul.

❧

Allergy:
Hist, Acon, Apis mel, Sulph.

Anaemia:
Ars alb, China, Nat mur, Ferr phos, Sil, Calc carb, Secale.

Anaesthesia recovery:
Too slow: Acetic ac, Phos
Too weak: Staph.
Too sore: Arnica.
Ice cold: Carbo veg.

Anger: (brooding)
Staph.

Anthrax: (esp cattle)
Ars alb, Lach, Echin, Pyro, Anthrac, Crot hor.

Anxiety: (anticipation)
Lyco, Arg nit.

Apathy:
China, Nat mur, Phos, Puls, Sep, Mur ac.
Appetite gone:
Calc carb, Nux v, Lyc, Puls, Rhus t, Nux v, Carbo veg.

Arthritis:
Arg nit, Bry, Puls, Rhod, Rhus t, Sulph, Apis m.

Asthma: (see Miasms)
Possibly Psor, Arsen alb.

Attention deficit:
Lach.

B.

Bad breath:
Carbo veg.
Fetid: Arnica, Merc sol.
Putrid: Aur met.
Carrion: Pyro.

Bites:
Ledum (dogbite), Lach, Golond, Guaco (Snake), Guaco (Scorpion), Indigo (Snake/Spider)
Flea and mosquito repellent: Caladium seg.

Bladder: (see urination)
Incontinent: Sep, Nat mur, Ignat, Calc fluor.
Retention: Acon, Canth, Lyco, Hyos, Cann sat.

Bleeding:
Ferr met, Phos (superficial).
Bright red blood: Bell.
Black blood: Both.
Vital Force dying: Carbo veg.
Persistent: China.
Oozing: Arnica.
Gushing red: Ipec, Ham.

Blisters:
Apis m, Rhus tox.

Bloat: (see abdominal distension)

Bad blood: (poisoning)
Hep sulph.

Blood poisoning:
Bell, Pyro, Bufo, Crot hor.

Body odour: (stink)
Sul.

Boils:
Ars alb, Graph, Hep sul, Sil.

Bones: (broken, swollen)
Symph, Calen, Ruta, Calc phos.

Bone infections:
Ruta, Symph, Calc phos.

Bruises:
Arnica, Hyper.
Internal: Bellis.
Easy bruisers: Phos.
Bruises stay black: Ledum, Sulph.
Bruised bone: Ruta.

Bronchitis:
Acon, Bry, Bell, Spong, Ars alb, Puls, Ledum, Beryl.

Broken wind: (horse)
Arsen alb.

Broodiness:
Ignatia.

Burns:
Urtica urens, Caust, Apis m, Canth.
Shock after burns: Acon.
To stop infection of burn: Arnica.
Prevent gangrene and scarring: Calen.

Scalds, blisters: Rhus tox.

❧

C

❧

Cancers: (see tumours)
Kreos, Therid cur, Coca.

❧

Car sickness: (motion, see travel)

❧

Catarrh:
Allium cep, Kali bich, Nat mur, Acon, Coccus, Hydras.

❧

Cataract: (see eye)

❧

Centipede attacks:
Apis m, Ledum.

❧

Chills:
Acon, Gels, Puls.
From wetness: Dulc.

❧

Cholera: (fowl)
Sore joints, lame: Rhus tox, Sulph.
No breath, nose blocked: Calc fluor and Hep sul, Kali bich.
Green diarrhoea: Puls, Sul.

Coccidiosis: (poultry)
Listless, blood in droppings: Ipec, Merc cor.
Pale comb no appetite: Chell, Nux v.
White head: Merc.

Colic: (gripes)
Mag phos, Coloc.
Cough: Dulc, Nux v, Squilla m, Amm mur, Dros, Puls.

Collapse: (complete)
Carbo veg.

Comb and wattles: (poultry)
Rose colour: China.

Concussion:
Arnica, Cic v, Rescue Remedy.

Conjunctivitis:
Acon, Arg nit, Euph, Rhus t.

Constipation:
Sil, Alum, Calc carb, Nit ac, Sep, Nux v, Lyco.

Cough: (see kennel cough)

Dry: Acon, Bell, Puls.
Wet: Ipec, Merc, Sep, Kali bich, Nat sul.
Spasmodic: Mag phos, Dros.
Tracheal infection: Bry.

Contortions:
Cic.

Convulsions:
Cic.

Cow –pox:
Cracks bleeding: Nux v.
Dry painful skin problems: Ant crud.
Yellow pus pimples: Kali bich.
Prominent pox on udder: Ranunc bulb
Prevention: Vario.

Cracks: (skin fissures)
Nit ac, Petro, Graph.

Cramp:
Mag phos.

Cuts:
Hyper.

Cystitis:
Sulph, Nux v, Ars alb, Arg nit.

❧

D.

❧

Dandruff:
Arsen alb, Sulph.

❧

Deafness:
China, Nit ac. Puls, Sil, Kali bich, Puls, Kali mur.

❧

Death and dying: (euthanasia)
Ars alb can ease death.
Fear of death: Acon.
Death Rattle: Ant-t.
Anguish of death: Arsen alb.
Stupid as if braindead: Opium.
Convulsions, cramps: Cup met.
Mania (uncontrolled activity): Tarent hisp.

❧

Debilitated: (see rundown)

❧

Delirium: (confusion)
Bell, Hyos, Stram, Ver alb, Phos, Agar.

❧

Depression: (discouraged)

Rescue Remedy, Ambra gris, Kali phos, Lyco, Onos.

De-hydration:
China.

Diarrhoea:
Arg nit, Ars alb, Bry.
Bad food: Ars alb, Ipec.
Eating from the garbage can: Nux v.
Stinking: Sulph.
Bloody: Phos. Trill.
Blood streaks or stains: Phos, Merc sol.
General: Podo.
From wet: Dulc.
Bad water: Arsen alb.
From stress or anticipatory anxiety: Arg nit.
From anti-biotics: Nit ac.
Green: Arg nit.

Distemper:(canine)
Distemp, Bapt, Ars alb.

Dizziness:(falls down) (esp horses)
Bell. Nux vom.
Faintness with dizziness: Trill.
Bleeding with dizziness: Trill.

E.

Ears:
Infection: Bell, Merc, Hep sulph, Pyro.
Violent pain: Chamo.
Acute pain: Hep sul.
Scaly and scabby: Kali bich.
Bloody discharge: Kali bich.
Stinking discharge: Merc sol/cor.
Thick yellow discharge: Lyc.
Hot red ears: Sulph.
Dry scaly: Arsen alb.
Dry cracks: Nat mur.
Sticky discharge: Graph.
Terrible itch and ulcer: Lyco.

Eczema: (see Skin, Miasms)

Edema:
Apis m.
Pulmonary: Ant t.

Electrocution:
Arnica, Phos.

Emphysema-like symptoms: (treat symptoms)
Ledum, Lob, Phos.

Epilepsy:
Ign, Bell, Rescue Remedy, Acon, Bufo.

❦

Excitement (too much):
Bell.

❦

Exhaustion:
Arnica, Kali phos.

❦

Eyes:
Euph, Allium Cepa.
Cataract: Cin mar.
Infection: Apis m, Merc cor, Thuja.
Lids: (paralysed) Gels.
Opaque: Euph, Cineraria.
Retina detached: Symph, Hama, Gels, Digit, Naphtha.
Trauma: Aconite.
Ulcers: Rhus t, Arg nit.
Edema (edema/puffiness): Apis m, Puls.

❦

F.

❦

Fatigue:
Arnica.

❦

Fears:
Gels, Arg nit, Ign, Lyco, Kali phos.

Of death: Acon.

⚜

Feathers always ruffled:
China sulph, Chell.

⚜

Feet: (birds-bumble foot)
CEH ointment (Calendula, Echinacea, Hypericum).

⚜

Fever:
Arsen.
Early stage: Acon.

⚜

Fits: (see convulsions):
Stram.

⚜

Fireworks: (fear of)
Gels.

⚜

Fleas: (see bites)
White dilute vinegar wash and 4 teaspoons vinegar in waterbowl regularly.

⚜

Fluid loss:
China.

⚜

Food poisoning: (see poisoning)
Ver alb, Carbo veg.

Foot rot:
Calc fluor, Hep sul, Sil, Nat mur.

Foreign bodies: (splinters etc)
Sil.

Frost bite:
Agar, Nux v.
Frozen: (hypothermia) Arsen alb, Vera alb.

Fur loss:
Arsen alb, Nat mur.
Rough fur no appetite: Ant crud.

G.

Gait:
Tripps stagger: Rhus tox.
Sluggish: Gels.
Staggering: Acon, Arg nit, Zinc.
Stumbling: Phos ac.
Trembling all over: Lact ac.

Gangrene:(threatening)
Arsen alb.
Dry: (toes etc) Secale.
Moist: Carbo veg.

✌

Giddiness:
Acon, Bella, Caust.
From old age: Rhus t, Sulph.

✌

Glands:
Jaborandi (Pilo mic), Hep sulph, Tuber, Calc fluor.

✌

Glanders:
Merc sol.

✌

Grief:
Aur m, Ign, Nat m, Puls.

✌

Growths: (see tumours)
Fungoid, bleeding: Phos, Thuja.

✌

Gums:
Merc sol, Apis mel.

✌

H.

✌

Haemorrhoids:
Aes, Sulph, Ham.
Bleeding constantly: Collin.
Protruding, bloody discharge: Merc viv after Thuja.
Fissures and burning: Nit ac.
Itches: Ant c.
Prolapse with sharp pain: Ignatia.
Protruding, strangulated with sphincter spasms, intense pain:
Hot poultice.

Haemorrhage: (internal)
Trill.

Hair ball:
Nux vom.

Hayfever:
Euph, All sep. Gels.

Head injury:
Arnica.
Delirious: Bella.
Unconscious/concussed: Cicuta v.
Fractures (skull), spasm, fits: Hyper.
Mental disturbance: Nat sulph.
Head bent back: Hyper.
Nerve damage: Hyper.

Head: swellings on bony parts:
Hekla lava.

❧

Head: black (birds):
Psor, Lach.

❧

Heart:
Acon, Arnica, Apis.
Palpitation: Aeth cyn, Cactus.

❧

Head blow, near death: (poultry)
Calc carb, Calc phos.

❧

Heatstroke:
Bella, Arnica, Acon, Vera alb.

❧

Hernia:
Nux v, Sulph.

❧

Herpes:
Rhus t, Pyro.

❧

Hiccoughs:
Nux v, Mag phos, Ipec, Ign.

❧

Homesickness: (kennels)
Ign, Nat mur.

❧

Horsefly bites:
Hyper.

❧

Hotspots:
White vinegar wash, Sulph.

❧

Hysteria:
Lach, Aur met, Ign, Gels.
Disproportionate reactions: Ign.
Loss of appetite, green/brown diarrhoea: Sulph, Ipec.

❧

I.

❧

Immune system:
Echinacea.

❧

Indigestion: (see abdominal distention)
Arg nit, Nux v, Puls, Sulph.

❧

Indifference:
Sepia.

❧

Infection: (severe)
Pyro, Lach.
Septic: Echin.
Puncture: Ledum.

Infertility:
Male: Agnus, Conium, Lyco, Sepia.
Female: Conium, Lyco, Sabina, Sepia.

Injury: (see wounds)

Interest: (gone, indifferent)
China, Puls, Sep, Phos, Nat mur.

Insomnia:
Coff, Opium, Ign, Gels, Cimif.

Itchy ears:
Sulph, Arsen alb.

Itches:
Anus: Alum, Nit ac, Sulph.
Dry, maddening, crawling, rectum esp: Teuc m.

J.

Jaundice:
Merc sol.

❧

Jerks (and **twitches** constantly):
Tarent Hisp, Agar, Zinc, Cim, Cup met.

❧

Joint pain:
Rhus t, Bry.

❧

K.

❧

Kennel cough: (see cough)
Dros rot, Bryonia.

❧

Kidney: (swelling, pain)
Apis m, Ars alb, Nat m, Bry.

❧

L.

❧

Lameness:
Lachesis, Nux Vomica, Bry.

❧

Leeches:
Lachesis.

❧

Lice on birds:
Sabad, Nux m, Sulph.

***

Lightning strike:
Nux v.

***

Liver: (enlarged esp birds)
Chell, China.
Jaundice: Merc sol.
Food caused: Nux v.
Chronic disease, swollen abdomen: Lyco.
Cancer of: Choles.

***

Lung: (emphysema)
Amm caust, Anti tart, Bry, Lobelia inf.
Coughing bloody mucus, cannot breathe: Acon, Ip, Mille, Ant t, Bry.

***

Lyme disease:
Ledum.

***

M.

***

Mange: (see Skin, Miasms)
Sulph, Arsen alb, Psor, Graph.

***

Mastitis:
Bell, Bry, Calc fluor.

Milk fever:
Acon, Bell, Mag phos, Opium, Phos, Cup met.
Milk production:
Too little: One dose Urtica, Puls, Cham, Caust.
Too much: Urtica 1c every six hours.

Mouth ulcers:
Hep sulph, Nit ac, Nat mur, Merc sol, Borax.

Muscular dystrophy: (esp poultry)
Brain: Kali phos, Calc phos, Sabina, Sepia.
Legs twisted: Acon, Calc phos.

N.

Nausea: (see vomiting)

Nervousness:
Arg nit, Ignatia, Lyco.
Weak, need support: Puls.

Newcastle disease:
Can't breathe: Acon, Ars alb.

Rattling cough: Ant t.
Paralysed legs: Kali phos, Calc phos, Gels.
Neck twisting: Mag phos, Sulph, Cicuta.

❧

Nipples: (teats)
Graphites (cracks and pain), Sil, Phyto, rub on Vaseline.

❧

Noise sensitivity:
Kali phos.

❧

Nose (discharges, blocked): (see catarrh)
Puls, Kali bich, Nat mur.

❧

O.

❧

Oil covered, cleaned:
Petroleum.

❧

Operations: (see surgery).

❧

Orchitis:
Hep sulph calc (pain), Apis mel, Puls, Clem, Rhod.

❧

P.

❧

Pain: (before storms)
Rhod.
After giving birth: Cimi, Cham, Puls, Gels.

❧

Panic, fear of death:
Acon.

❧

Paralysis:
Old age: Baryta c.
Panic: Ign.
Rigid: Strych.
Slow or throat: Gels.
Throat and mouth: Lath sat.
Nerve damage: Hyper.
Single parts: (also bladder, larynx, pharynx) Caust.
Front legs: Plum met.
Rear legs: Conium, Pic ac.
In chickens: Caust.
Progressive Spinal: Phos, Alum, Rhus tox.
Eyelids: Gels.
Motor system: Curare, Lath sat.
Ascending sensory and motor paralysis from paws up: Phos.
General: Suggest dosing with combination 12 Tissue
Salts.

❧

Parasites:
Gut pain, ascarides: Indigo.

Intestine: Aconite

Parvo virus:
Enteric form: Acon, Nux vom, Ars alb, Merc sol,
Cardiac form: Apis, Digitalis, Caroteus.

Piles: (see Haemorrhoids)
Nit ac, Hyper.

Poisoning: (dose hourly or more frequently until improvement then slow down)
Food: Ars alb, Carbo veg, Coloc.
Acids: Caust, Canth.
Detergents: Lach.
Petroleum products: Petro, Ipecac.
Lead: Plum.
Aluminium: Alum.
Bad fish: China.
Bad water: Arsen alb, Bapt, Zing.
Rat poison: Arsen alb, Ip, Merc, Phos, Verat.
Kreosote: Kreos.
Strychnine rodent poisons: Nux v, Cham.
Turps: Nux v.
Warfarin (bleeding): Trill, Crot hor, Mille.

Pox (virus):
Ant crud, Vario.
Pox: Fowl (with spots) Ant t.
Growth warts in mouth: Kali m, Kali sulph.

With high temp: Acon.
With no temp: Bry, Calc phos.
Head only: Vario.

Pneumonia:
Acon, Ant t, Bry, Lyco, Stan met, Tuber, Beryl.

Pregnancy (false):
Vicious patient: Sep.
Milk: Puls.

Prolapse (body-part falling out of its place):
Thuja, Podo.
Uterus: Calc phos, Carbo veg, Sepia, Podo, Lil tig.
In birds: Ferr phos, Kali mur, Calc fluor.
Rectum: Ruta, Sulph, Podo, Nux v.

R.

Rabies: (booster reaction)
Lyssin (Hydroph).

Rage:
Staph.

Respiratory Disease:

(*Esp cats*): Puls, Arsen alb, Merc viv/sol.

Chronic Respiratory Disease (CRD) air sac disease in birds especially broilers (see sneezing, eyes, nose).

Early stage: Acon.

Lungs blocked: Ant t.

Short breath: Phos.

Distress when moving: Beryl.

❧

Restlessness:

Rhus t, Arsen alb, Arg nit.

❧

Rheumatism:

Rhus t, Bry, Ruta, Calc c, Sulph.

❧

Ring (showring): (fear of shows)

Gels, Arg nit.

❧

Ringworm: (advanced, crusty)

Sep, Baccil, Tell, Chrys, Psor, Dulc, Sulph.

❧

Rubbing: (see touch)

❧

Rundown: (debilitated)

Nux v, Kali phos, Calc carb, Ars alb, Arn, Sep.

❧

S.

Sadness:
Lach.

Septicaemia:
Lach, Ars alb, Echin, Pyro.

Shock:
Acon, Arnica, Ars, Carbo veg, Rescue remedy.

Skin: (ulceration, see Eczema and Mange)
Arsen alb, Sil, Nit ac, Lach, Bell.
Dry, greasy, yukky: Graph.
Abrasions: Cal, Hyper.
See Miasms.

Snakebite: (see bites)
Lach, Apis m, Bell, Ledum.

Sneezing:
Amm phos.

Solitude: (craving for full time)
Sep.

Spasms:
Mag phos, Passi.

Spinal injury:
Bone damage: Symph.
Damage: Hyper.
Sprains and strains: Ruta, Acon, Arn, Rhus t.
Head (neck) twisted sideways: Cic vir.

Stiffness:
Arnica, Bry, Ruta, Berb vul, Phyto.
Easing with motion: Rhus t.

Stings:
Apis m, Bell, Ledum.
Wasp: Vespa crab.

Stinking body and discharges:
Sulph.

Storms: (fear of)
Rhod, Nat m.

Strangles:
Merc sol, Sulph.

Sunstroke:
Merc sol, Arsen alb, Caust, Urt u, Glon, Bella.

Sulking: (prolonged)
Ignatia.

Surgery:
Arnica.
Before: Arn.
After: Arnica, Acon, Bellis, China, Hyper, Ledum.
Aid after: Kali phos.
Constipation after: Nux v.

Swallowing: (obstructed feeling)
China, Gels, Ign, Lach, Nit ac.

Swelling:
(Rapid): Bell.
(Slow): Apis m.
Feet and Leg joints: (especially birds) Acon, Rhus t.

T.

Teething:
Chamo.

Terror: (see Panic, Fear)
Acon, Arg nit, Ign.

Tetanus:
Rigidity: Strych, Cup met (blue), Ledum, Hyper.
Convulsions: Nux v, Cic, Physo, Stram.
Horses, hot countries: Passi (large doses).

Thunder terror:
Gels.

Tongue:
Merc hyd.
Yellow: Bry.
Black cracked: Ars alb.
Red tip: Rhus tox.
Blue: (esp cows) Acon, Nat mur, Ars alb, Rhus t, Merc.
Flabby with teeth marks: Merc sol.
In and out like a snake: Cup met.

Touch: (aversion to)
Arn.
Piercing pain when touched: Bry.
Pain eased by touch: Rhus tox.

Travel sickness:
Acon, Gels, Petro.

Trembling:
Kali phos, Rhus t.

❦

Tuberculosis: (treat symptoms)
Tuber.

❦

Tumours: (suspected malignant)
Kali phos.
On ovaries heart, kidneys: (especially poultry), Calc fluor,
Phyto.
  Pains of: Silicea.
  Spongy: Hekla lava.
  Of glands: Conium.
  Fatty: Baryta c.
  Uterus: Iod.

❦

Twitches: (see jerks)

❦

Typhoid-like symptoms: (treat symptoms)
Typh.

❦

U.

❦

Ulcers on skin: (foul smelling)
Merc hyd.

❦

Umbilical infection:
Strep, Pyro, Abro.

Unconscious:
Carbo veg, Digi, Can ind.

Urinary problems: (cystitis)
Bell, Apis m, Canth.
Bloody urine after exercise: Can ind.
Violent strain to urinate: Can ind.

V.

Vaccinosis:
Reaction to vaccination: Thuja.
Fear of water plus aggression/rage: Lyssin (Hydro).
Vaginal discharge: Puls, Bell.

Vomitting:
Ipec, Cup met, Ars alb, Nux v.
With violent retching: Tabac.

W.

Warts:
Thuja, Calc carb.
Flat warts on teats: Caust.

Large flat warts on head and limbs: Dulc.
Bleeding warts: Ac nit.
Genital warts: Sabina.
Ulcers round warts: Ars alb.

Wax in ears, blocked, red, stinking:
Psor, Con m.

Weakness:
Bov, China sulph, Kali phos.

Wheezing, no air:
Arsen alb.

Wounds:
Arn, Hyper, Phos.

Worms: (see parasites)
China, Calad, Cic, Spig, Ign, Sab, Calc.
Pinworms: Teuc, Sinap nig.

Y.

Yawning:
Nux vom, Rhus t, China, Tarent hisp.

Materia Medica for the First Response.

Abrotanum (Abro, Southernwood, Artemisia Abrotanum).

Lower extremities, rheumatism, diarrhoea, suppressed conditions, TB, pleurisy, haemorrhoids.

Mind: Irritable, angry, depressed.

Stomach: Food passes undigested, gnawing pains worse at night, vomitting.

Abdomen: Ascarides, distension, diarrhoea and constipation alternating.

Respiration: Difficulty, dry cough.

Back: Pains, neck so weak head hangs and flops.

Extremities: Pains everywhere, stiff and lame, limbs emaciated.

Skin: Eruptions, purple, flabby, furuncles.

Worse: Cold, checked emissions.

Better: Motion.

Acetic acid (Acet ac, Glacial Acetic Acid).

Anaemia, dropsy, debility, weak heart, vomitting, profuse urination and sweat, wasting.

Mind: Irritable, worried.

Head: Blood rushes.

Stomach: Fermented, vomitting, sour belching, profuse salivation.

Abdomen: Bowel haemorrhage, frequent watery stools.
Urine: Pale, profuse, diabetes.
Female: Enlarged teats, impoverished milk, bleeding after labour, anaemia.
Respiration: Coarse, hissing, difficult, rattle.
Back: Pain relieved by lying on abdomen.
Extremities: Edema of legs and feet.
Skin: Hot, dry, varicose, burning, scurvy.
Fever: Profuse, no thirst.
Antidotes all anaesthetic vapours.

Aconitum Napellus (Monkshood).

Fear, anguish, restlessness, sudden violent invasion of disease, weakness, fever, action brief and effective at the onset.
Mind: Fear of death!
Head: Bursting, sometimes delirious.
Eyes: Swollen, red, averse to light or brightness.
Ears: Hot, red, averse to noise. Earache.
Nose: Coryza, sneezing, running, blocked.
Mouth: Tongue swollen, gums inflamed, jaw constantly in motion.
Throat: Red, dry, constricted.
Stomach: Vomitting, terrible thirst, about to die.
Abdomen: Tight like drum, painful to touch.
Rectum: Painful, stool green like chopped spinach, bleeding piles.
Urine: Burning, red hot, suppressed, bloody, retention, screaming.
Male: Crawling, stinging pain, swollen hard testicles.
Female: Stabbing pain in ovaries.
Respiration: Difficult with hacking cough.
Heart: Palpitations.

Back: Pains, stiff.
Extremities: Pains, lameness, unsteadiness.
Sleep: Terrible dreams.
Skin: Red hot, dry rash.
Fever: Coldness with thirst.
Better: In open air, worse in warmth.

Aesculus Hippocastanum (Aes, Horse Chestnut).
Lower bowel, haemorrhoidal veins, painful but little bleeding, venous problems, purple veins, congested system, pains, swollen dry membranes, throat.
Head: Pain, confusion, nausea.
Eyes: Painful red-veined, watery.
Nose: Dry, sneezy, runny.
Mouth: Salivating, coated tongue.
Throat: Raw, dry, struggle to swallow.
Stomach: Pain, sensitive.
Rectum: Raw, painful, prolapse, piles, large hard stool, burning.
Urine: Hot, dark, a little often.
Chest: Coughs and panting.
Extremities: Aching pains.
Back: Lame neck, sore feet, back and legs collapse.

Aethusa Cynapium (Aeth cyn, Fool's Parsley).
Brain and nervous system affected, diarrhoea, inability to digest milk, circulation problems, sudden onset.
Mind: Restless, idiocy, brain fag (not regenerating), crazy.
Head: Vertigo, palpitations, drowsiness, relieved by stomach expelling gas.

Eyes: Rolling, dilated, photophobia.
Ears: Uncomfortable.
Nose: Blocked completely.
Mouth: Pustules in throat, difficulty swallowing.
Stomach: Vomits then wants food, distress.
Stool: Undigested, green, constipated.
Urinary: Pains in bladder and kidneys.
Female: Lancinating pains, itching pimples.
Respiration: Very difficult, voiceless with hardship, cramps.
Heart: Palpitation.
Extremities: Numb, weak, spasms.
Skin: Itchy eruptions, swollen lymph glands.
Fever: Great heat no thirst.
Sleep: Great startling in sleep.
Better: Open air, company.

&

Agaricus Muscarius-Amanita (Agar, Toad Stool, Bug Agaric).
Slow acting, brain intoxicant followed by stupor, vertigo. Jerks, twitches, anaemia, spasms, cerebral effervescence, violent pains, worse for touch and cold.
Mind: Noisy, indifferent, fearless, yawns. Excitement grows in phases.
Head: Moves constantly, falls around.
Eyes: Twitching, red.
Ears: Burn and itch, twitchings.
Nose: Itching, sneezing, coughing.
Mouth: Great thirst, quivering white tongue.
Throat: A struggle to swallow, dry.
Stomach: Distended, flatulent.
Abdomen: Diarrhoea with flatus. Pains under ribs, odorous stool.

Urination: Sudden compulsions, frequent.
Female: Itches, pain, burning.
Respiratory: Violent coughing, struggle to breathe.
Heart: Palpitating.
Extremities: Stiff all over, gait affected, pains.
Skin: Burning, itching, red, swollen veins, hotspots.
Fever: Violent fevers in evening.
Worse: Cold air, open air, eating, storms.
Better: For slow moving.

Agnus Castus (Ag cas, The Chaste Tree).
Attacks on sexual organs, loss of nerve power, premature ageing, itch, weakened heart.
Mind: Fearful, forgetful, sad.
Eyes: Itches, photophobia, dilations.
Abdomen: Sore swellings, anal fissures.
Male: Discharges, cold, pains.
Female: Discharge, sterility, nose bleeds, heart palpitations.

Aletris Farinosa (Alet far, Stargrass root).
Anaemic, relaxed, female, tired, prolapses.
Mind: Confused, weak, no energy.
Mouth: Froth.
Stomach: Distress, vertigo, flatulence, dyspepsia.
Stool: Large, hard, painful.
Female: Prone to abortions, weak.

Allium Cepa (Al cep, Red Onion).
Runny acrid discharge nose and eyes, larynx, burning, red.

Ears: Shooting pains.
Nose: Sneezing, hayfever, cough, discharge, wet.
Stomach: Hunger, thirst, belching, nausea.
Abdomen: Rumbling, odorous gas.
Rectum: Itching, glowing heat, offensive flatus, diarrhoea.
Urination: Pain, red.
Respiration: Hacking cough, pain.
Extremities: Lame, pains, soreness, tired feeling.
Worse: Warmth.
Better: Cold air.

Alumina (Oxide of Aluminium–Argilla).
Dry mucous membranes and skin, sluggish system, debilitated, constipated.
Mind: Poor spirits.
Head: Hairloss, itches, pain, vertigo.
Eyes: Conjunctivitis.
Ears: Partly deaf.
Nose: Red, painful, coryza.
Face: Lower jaw twitches.
Mouth: Stinking, sore gums, bleeding.
Throat: Cannot swallow.
Stomach: Aversion to meat, great discomfort, no hunger.
Abdomen: Colic.
Stool: Hard, dry, pain, difficulty, diarrhoea with urination.
Urination: Straining.
Respiration: Cough, wheezing, rattling, tickle, pain.
Back: Pain, paralytic weakness.
Extremities: Pain, burning, paralysis, staggering, sore, swollen, spinal degeneration.

Sleep: Restless.
Skin: Scratching until it bleeds.
Worse: Morning, waking, warmth.
Better: Open air, cold water, evening, damp.

Ambra Grisea (Ambra gris, Morbid Secretion of the Whale).
Excitable, nervous, thin, anaemic, sleepless, one-sided complaints, parts, weakness, exhaustion, aggravated by music.
Mind: Seeks solitude.
Head: Poor hearing, slow, vertigo, tearing pain, depression, dizziness.
Stomach: Distension, convulsive coughing.
Urination: Painful, dark sediment.
Female: Great itching.
Male: Violent itches of the scrotum.
Respiration: Difficulty, hollow barking cough, tickling throat, out of breath when coughing.
Heart: Palpitation.
Sleep: Disturbed.
Skin: Itchy and sore especially round genitals.
Extremities: Cramps everywhere and anywhere.

Ammonium Causticum (Amm caust, Hydrate of Ammonia – Ammonia Water).
Cardiac stimulant, snake bite, bleeding, thrombosis, oedema, ulceration of mucus membrane.
Respiration: Difficult, clogged with mucus, gasping, burning discharge.
Extremities: Rheumatism, exhaustion, debility, hot dry skin.

Ammonium Muriaticum (Amm mur, Sal Ammoniac).

Prostration, fat and sluggish, struggle to breathe, irregular circulation, coughs, profuse secretions.

Head: Itching, dandruff, hairloss.

Eyes: Cataracts pending, poor vision.

Nose: Acrid, runny, itchy, no smell, sore to touch, sneezing.

Throat: Can hardly swallow, pain, constriction.

Stomach: Cancer, nausea, vomitting up food.

Abdomen: Pain, congested liver, flatus, fat round abdomen.

Rectum: Itching piles, green stools, burning, sometimes constipated.

Respiration: Cough, chest rattles, salivation, dry hacking.

Extremities: Neuralgia and pains.

Skin: Itching blisters.

Better: Open air.

Worse: Mornings.

Ammonium Phosphoricum (Amm phos, Phosphate of Ammonia).

Gout, uric acid, bronchitis, sore joints, facial paralysis, chest and shoulder pains, wobbly gait, unsteady.

Head: Sneezing, excessively runny eyes and nose in mornings.

Respiratory: Deep cough with green phlegm.

Urine: Sediment, pink.

Antimonium Arsenicosum (Ant ars, Arsenite of Antimony).

Emphysema, cough, mucus, pneumonia, weak heart, facial edema, red eyes, weakness.

Antimonium Crudum (Anti crud, Black Sulphide of Antimony).

Irritability, coated white tongue, hates the sun, no appetite, unhappy digestive system.

Mind: Grumpy, peevish.

Eyes: Blepharitis, dull, red, fissured, pustules.

Nose: Scurfy, exzema, crusts.

Face: Yellow pus boils and pimples.

Mouth: Dry lips, cracks, raw palate, gum problems, sores, exzema.

Throat: Yellow mucous running down back.

Stomach: Vomitting, sour, belching, bloat.

Stool: Diarrhoea alternates with constipation, slimy flatulent stools with watery discharges, mucus oozing.

Urine: Burning, stinking.

Male: Atrophy or organs.

Female: Itchy.

Respiratory: Coughs.

Back: Itching and pains.

Skin: Eczema, warts, urticaria, growths, burns, itches.

Antimonium Tartaricum (Anti tar, Tartar Emetic, Tartrate of Antimony and Potash).

Respiratory, rattling mucus, drowsy, debilitated, catarrhs of the entire system, mucus stools, Bilharziasis, trembling, muscular pains, genital warts.

Mind and head: Downhearted, vertigo, so tired.
Tongue: Coated, white with red sides, dry in centre.
Face: Quivering lower jaw.
Stomach: Vomitting, nausea, retching, thirst.
Abdomen: Pressure, colic, bloat, diarrhoea.
Urine: Blood, pain, orchitis.
Respiration: Mucus, trouble breathing, cough, partial paralysis of the lungs, palpitation, weak pulse.
Back: Pain, tremble, retching when moves.
Skin: Pus pimples, warts, growths, pox.
Fever: Intense.
Sleep: Tired, exhausted, jerks and twitches.
Worse: Evening, lying.
Better: Up and about.

❧

Apis Mellifica (Apis m, Honey-bee).
Edema of skin and mucus membranes. Swellings, puffiness, rosy, stinging, sore to touch, dropsy. Outer skin of organs or skin primarily, inflammation. Stiffness, prostration.
Mind: No interest, disturbed, unhappy.
Head: Tired, sneezing, dull, shrieks.
Eyes: Swollen, hot, red, styes.
Ears: Red, inflamed, sore.
Nose: Red, swollen, cold on end.
Face: Swollen, stinging, puffy.
Mouth: Red, swollen raw tongue, sores in mouth and throat.
Stomach: No thirst, vomitting.
Abdomen: Tender.
Stool: Raw, holds in nothing, diarrhoea, dark, horrible, constipation sometimes.
Urine: Stinging, incontinent.

Female: Sore, tender, stinging.
Respiratory: Suffocating, throat swollen.
Extremities: Joints swollen, sore, hives, itches.
Skin: Swellings, rosy, sensitive, body puffy.
Sleep: Disturbed.
Fever: Comes and goes.
Worse: Any touch.

Argentum nitricum (Arg nit, Nitrate of Silver).
Brain and spine, co-ordination, flatulence, premature ageing, anaemia.
   Mind: Hurried, fears, anxiety, wants to stay at home.
   Head: Brain fag, debility, nervous.
   Eyes: Swollen, red, discharge, no steady gaze, opaque.
   Nose: Itchy, ulcers, coryza.
   Mouth: Red tipped, gums painful, sores in mouth.
   Throat: Raw, coughing, mucus, hawking.
   Stomach: Nausea, vomitting, flatulence, distension.
   Abdomen: Distended, painful.
   Stool: Green, shreddy, disgusting, flatulence, fluids, itching.
   Urine: Bloody, oozes, painful, stream can be divided.
   Male: Genitals shrivelled.
   Respiratory: Cough, suffocating, pain in chest.
   Back: Pain in spine.
   Extremities: Weak, paralysed, rigid, unsteady.
   Skin: Hard, withered, blotched, dried.
   Worse: Warmth.
   Better: Cold air, pressure.

Arnica (Arn, Leopard's Bane).

Any injury, overuse, exhaustion, trauma, pain, bruise, heart condition, surgery.

Mind: Fears, fear of touch, of approach.

Head: Not right.

Eyes: Muscular paralysis, bleeding.

Ears: Pains inside.

Nose: Bleeds, sore.

Mouth: Stinks, bad gums and sore teeth.

Stomach: Hunger, vomitting, pain, gas, discomfort.

Abdomen: Distended, unpleasant flatus.

Stool: Pain, strain, offensive, bloody.

Female: After labour, with any problems.

Respiration: Pneumonia, coughs, pains, spasms, whooping.

Heart: Weak pulse, pain.

Extremities: Fear of touch, pain everywhere, gait affected, rheumatism.

Skin: Acne, spots, pimples, sores.

Sleep: Soils bed, terrible dreams, disturbance.

Fever: Shivering heat.

ح‌ه

Arsenicum album (Arsen alb, Arsenious Acid, Arsenic Trioxide).

Affects every organ and tissue. Debility, exhaustion, restlessness, nightly aggravation, burning relieved by heat, fear, poison, stings, stink and degeneration, anaemia, low vitality, septic situations, green discharge.

Mind: Fear, disturbed.

Head: Cold skin, burning heat, relieved by cold, constant motion, delirium, itches, scales.

Ears: Raw inside, pain, stink.

Nose: Running, burning, bleeding.

Mouth: Tongue dry, red, gum problems, bloody saliva, gulping of water with pain.

Throat: Cannot swallow.

Stomach: Vomit, green bile, nausea, retching, cannot swallow, averse to food.

Abdomen: Terrible pain, distension, coughing.

Rectum: Burning pain. Prolapse. Skin excoriating (open wound).

Stool: Bloody, offensive, awful diarrhoea.

Urine: Pus and blood, involuntary.

Respiratory: Suffocates when lying down, asthma, catarrh, dry cough.

Back: Pain.

Extremities: Cramp, swollen feet, diabetic gangrene, ulcers, paralysis, atrophy.

Skin: Itching burning eruptions, gangrene, foul smell, offensive ulcers with vile discharge.

Sleep: Terrible suffering, suffocating, dreams.

Fevers: Intense, exhausting.

Aurum Metallicum (Aurum met, Metallic Gold).

Blood, glands, bone, tissue degeneration, body fluids, depression, pain, head pains, palpitation, congestion, paroxysms of pain in chest, sclerosis of liver, arteries, brain, lifeless, no joy.

Mind: Deranged.

Head: Vertigo, pains, boils.

Eyes: Photophobia.

Ears: Infection, pus, labyrinthitis (dizziness).

Nose: Ulcerated, stinking discharge, bloody, knobby end.

Mouth: Gums rotten.

Abdomen: Swollen, flatulent.

Urine: Retention, painful with sediment, thick.
Rectum: Constipation, burning.
Male: Pain.
Female: Enlarged, prolapsed.
Heart: Rapid beat.
Bones: Breaking down, great pain.
Extremities: Weakness, terrible pains.
Sleep: Disturbed.
Worse: Cold, winter.

Bacillinus (Bacill, Maceration of a Tuberculous Lung).

Chronic respiratory disease, lungs, catarrh, suffocation, constant chills.

Head: Ringworm, depression, red eyelids.

Abdomen: Constipation, diarrhoea, bloat.

Respiratory: Bubbling congestion of lungs, catarrh, expectoration.

Skin: Eczema, ringworm, fungus, pityriasis (itches).

Baryta Carb (Baryta c, Carbonate of Baryta).

For underdeveloped or slow developing creatures, sickly, unhealthy, not robust, weak in structure, or degenerative bodies and minds, glands, gums, internal organs, arteries, extremities, heart and muscle problems.

Mind: Timid, no drive, afraid of strangers.

Head: Confused.

Eyes: Cataracts, photophobia, pupils alternately dilating and contracting.

Ears: Poor hearing.

Nose: Thick yellow discharge, sneezing, bleeding, crusts.

Face: Top lip enlarged.

Mouth: Gums bleeding and pulled back, salivating, oesophageal spasm on swallowing, tongue paralysed.

Throat: Raw, painful to swallow, can take liquids but solids cause choking.

Stomach: Hiccough, eructation, hungry but cannot eat.

Abdomen: Rock hard, painful, colic.

Rectum: Protruding piles, crawling itches, large hard stools.

Urine: Piles protrude when urinating, burns.

Respiratory: Dry weak cough, suffocating.

Heart: Racing beat.

Back: Spine weak.

Extremities: Pains in lower limbs, joints sore.

Baptista (Bapt, Wild Indigo).

Septic blood conditions, sick, putrification, all discharges disgusting, anti-typhoid in humans.

Mind: Confusion.

Head: Stupor, deafness, vertigo.

Mouth: Teeth and gums sore and loose, stinking breath, ulcerated, tongue dark yellow, brown in centre and red on edges, cracks, cannot eat solids.

Throat: Stinks, cannot take food, painless, constricted and contracted, red.

Stomach: Vomitting.

Belladonna (Bell, Deadly Nightshade).

Nervous and vascular systems, excitement, convulsions, skin, glands, delirium, epilepsy, nausea, vomitting, scarlet fever symptoms, goitre, airsickness, sudden violent attack.

Mind: Crazed in the head, terrible images in mind, eyes do not function.

Head: Vertigo, throbbing pain, laboured breath with heart palpitations throbbing in head, cannot be touched, falls to the left or backward, moans with agony.

Face: Convulsive twitching, constant movement.

Eyes: Protruding, photophobia, spasms of lids, swollen lids.

Ears: Delirium from the pain, echoing inside head.

Nose: Red, swollen, bleeding, coryza.

Mouth: Gumboils, red swollen tongue, throbbing pain.

Throat: Raw, red, infested, swollen, tries to swallow all the time.

Stomach: Nausea, vomitting, retching, aversion to food and drink.

Abdomen: Hot, swollen, cannot be touched.

Stool: Thick green, prolapse, piles, shuddering with searing pains.

Urine: Thick and dark, incontinent, frequent and profuse.

Female: Tumours and revolting discharges.

Respiratory: Hacking, barking, painful cough.

Heart: Palpitates wildly.

Extremities: Swollen red shiny joints with red streaks, wobbly gait, limping, spasms, jerks.

Skin: Eruptions, pustules, boils, suppurating wounds, inflammations.

Bellis Perennis (Bell per, Daisy, Marguerite).

Muscles and blood vessels, lameness, venous congestion, deep injury, severe pain in nerves, intolerance of cold, sprains, bruises, boils, rheumatism, for old and tired bodies.

Head: Vertigo.

Abdomen: Diarrhoea, yellow and painless, terrible stench, bloat, rumbling.

Skin: Exudations, boils, swellings, painful to the touch.

Extremities: Painful muscles and joints, itches, sprains.

Berberis Vulgaris (Berb v, Barberry).

Symptoms changing to their opposites (e.g. raging thirst switches to aversion to water), rheumatism, haemorrhoids, urinary, pains all over, stones kidney and gall, liver, bile, spine.

Head: No interest in anything.

Nose: Left nostril blocked, troublesome.

Mouth: Sticky saliva.

Abdomen: Constipation, pains.

Stool: Yellow diarrhoea, tearing round anus.

Urine: Red with sand and thick mucus, frequent with burning.

Respiratory: Laryngeal polyps, pain.

Back: Lumbago.

Extremities: Rheumatism, joints and underfoot pain, lame, weary.

Skin: Pustules, itches, eczema, burning, flat warts.

Worse: Moving.

Beryllium Metallicum (Beryl m).

Lungs, eyes, skin, liver, kidneys, heart, nervous system, lymphatic system-white blood cells and proteins.

Eyes: Inflamed, in association with dermatitis.

Nose and throat: Inflammation, swelling.

Skin: Itching, redness, rashes, swelling, blisters, lesions, ulcers and little growths, wounds cannot heal.

Respiratory system: Coughing, weakness, tiredness, loss of appetite, weight loss, pneumonitis (air sac infection), possibly death.

Lesions: Toxicity causes granulomas (tissue masses like growths), on lungs, skin, liver, spleen, bone, nervous system, muscles, lymph glands and heart wall.

Borax (Bor, Borate of Sodium).

Gastric disorders, ulceration of mucus membranes, skin problems, delirium, diarrhoea, collapse, nausea, vomitting, colic (gut spasms), epilepsy.

Mind: Fear of noise, thunder and motion.

Head: Nausea with trembling.

Eyes: Lids red, lashes turned inward, eyes, scratched.

Ears: Very averse to small noises.

Nose: Swollen, ulcerated, red, shiny, swollen.

Face: Looks ill.

Mouth: Bleeding ulcers, gumboils, white fungous inside.

Stomach and abdomen: Distended, vomitting.

Stool: Offensive diarrhoea, colic.

Urine: Hot, burning, painful, smelly, red spots in it.

Female: Itches, sterility.

Respiratory: Hacking cough, bad smell, breathless on movement.

Extremities: Itches, pains, stitches, inflammation, eczema, nails fall off.

Skin: Itches, suppuration, eruptions.

Bothrops Lanciolatus (Both Lan, Bothrops, Lachesis Lanciolatus, Yellow Viper venom).

Thrombosis (blood clot), coagulated, septic, sluggish, broken down, tongue will not function properly, chest congestion, haemorrhages from all orifices.

Eyes: Haemorrhage into retina, blindness, conjunctival (eye) haemorrhage.

Face: Stupid expression.

Throat: Dry, constricted, unable to swallow liquids easily.

Stomach: As tight as a drum, bloody stool, black vomit.

Skin: Gangrenous, livid, haemorrhagic.

Bovista (Bov, Puff-Ball).

Skin eruptions, poor circulation, bleeding, exhaustion, asphyxia.

Head: Nasal discharge, dumb mind, itches.

Face: Nostrils and mouth crusty, bleeding nose and gums.

Abdomen: Red urine, colic.

Extremities: Clumsy, weary, itches.

Skin: Urticaria, itches, crusts, pimples, scurvy, eruptions.

Bryonia (Bry, Wild Hops).

Mucous membranes in viscera, dryness, irritability, excessive thirst, vertigo, constipation, puffiness, tearing pains everywhere.

Mind: Irritable, delirium.

Head: Vertigo, nausea, pain.

Nose: Coryza.

Eyes: Pain for touch or moving.

Mouth: Lips dry, black, thirst, tongue yellow/brown with white cover.

Throat: Dry, cannot swallow, sticky mucus.

Stomach: Distention after eating, vomitting of bile and water, excessive thirst and hunger.

Abdomen: Liver area swollen and sore.

Stool: Constipation, bloody stools.

Urine: Reddish brown, hot.

Respiratory: Dry hacking cough, vomit, difficulty breathing.

Extremities: Swollen sore joints, painful to touch, left side may move rhythmically.

Skin: Greasy, puffy, hot, pale.

Bufo (Poison of the Toad).

Derangements of the mind, seizures, feeble-mindedness, rheumatic symptoms, nervous system and skin disorders.

Mind: Feeble-minded, bites, howls, nervous.

Head: Nosebleed.

Eyes: Cannot take brightness, little blisters on eye.

Ears: Even small noises distress greatly.

Heart: Palpitation.

Extremities: Pains, cramps, staggering, swelling of bones.

Skin: Pustules, suppuration, blisters, itches, burning, carbuncles.

Cactus Grandiflorus (Cactus, Selenicereus Spinulosis, Night-blooming Cereus).

Heart and arteries, constrictive fibres, bladder, spasms, constrictions, panting and collapse.

Mind: Screams with pain, out of humour, anxious.

Head: Pain all over, periodically, poor hearing.

Nose: Bleeding, running.

Throat: Too dry cannot swallow food, constricted, suffocating.

Stomach: Vomits blood.

Stool: Painful piles, bleeding, hard black stool, diarrhoea mornings.

Urine: Tries constantly, bloody, turbid.

Female: Constant pain.

Chest: Convulsive painful cough, difficulty breathing.

Heart: Problematic, palpitations, irregular beat, murmers.

Extremities: Enlarged, puffy, cold, fidgety especially in sleep.

Sleep: Night terrors and wakefulness.

Fevers: Same time daily, coldness, anguish.

Caladium Seguinum (Calad, American Arum).

Genitals, single parts of body, motion aversion, asthma, heart.

Mind: Confusion, forgetful, hates noise, sore ears.

Stomach: Eructations, vomitting, sighing, cannot take deep breaths.

Male: Itches, discomfort.

Skin: Burning itches, flies attracted.

Respiratory: Asthma, constrictions, catarrh.

Calcarea Carbonica-Ostrearum (Calc carb, Carbonate of Lime).

Impaired nutrition, digestion, glands, skin, bones, coughs, breathlessness, abscesses, polyps, generally weak, not normal.

Mind: Fearful, confused.

Head: Vertigo, itches on head.

Eyes: Cataract, itchy, red, photophobia, ulcers on cornea, tears, lids swollen and scurfy.

Ears: Polyps, poor hearing, sensitive.

Nose: Ulcerated, dry, sore, yellow discharge, odour, coryza.

Mouth: Bleeding gums sore teeth, bad smell.

Throat: Difficult swallowing.

Stomach: Ravenous hunger, thirsty, averse to meat, eructations, belching, milk causes problems, swollen stomach disc-shaped swelling, worse for eating.

Abdomen: Swollen hard, flatulent, sore to the touch, trembling.

Stool: Crawling itches, hard stool, sour smell, prolapse, haemorrhoids, constipation and diarrhoea.

Urine: Profuse, bloody, with sediment, fetid, dark brown.

Female: Burning, itching, too much or too little milk.

Respiratory: Cough, blood, suffocation, cannot be touched must have fresh air.

Heart: Night palpitation and after eating.

Back: Rheumatic pains and weakness, rigid neck.

Extremities: Rheumatic pains, cramp, swollen joints, sores under pads.

Sleep: Very disturbed, terrors.

Fever: Same times daily.

Skin: Suppuration, itches, boils, warts, ulcers.

Calcarea Phosphorica (Calc phos, Phosphate of Lime).

Tissue remedy, bones, breaks, anaemia, wasting disease, diseased glands and organs.

Mind: Restless, irritable.

Head: Pain, poor hearing, hot with abdominal flatulence.

Eyes: Abscesses, opacity.

Mouth: Painful to open, rotten teeth, swollen throat.

Stomach: Hunger and thirst, eructations.

Abdomen: Flabby, retracted, colic, pains round navel.

Stool: Bleeding after large hard stools, hot sputtering green diarrhoea with gas.

Urine: Plentiful.

Female: Prolapses.

Respiratory: Suffocating and sighing, coughing.

Back and neck: Rheumatic.

Extremities: Joint and bone pain, stiff.

Calcarea Sulphurica (Calc sulph, Sulphate of Lime, Plaster of Paris).

Glands, skin, tumours, fibroids, suppurations with thick yellow pus.

Head: Yellow crusts on skin.

Eyes: Inflamed with yellow discharge, slightly opaque.

Ears: Discharge with blood, deaf, pimples.

Nose: Bloody, thick, yellow, stinking discharge, sometimes one-sided, raw nostrils.

Mouth: Flabby clay tongue with yellow-coated base.

Throat: Ulcerated, suppurating.

Abdomen: Pain, nausea.

Stool: Bloody diarrhoea, slimy pus discharge, abscesses round anus.

Respiratory: Cough, lungs full of pus, catarrh thick and lumpy.

Extremities: Burning and itching under paws.

Skin: Pus from every tiny wound, yellow discharge, crusts, yellow scabs, bleeding easily.

Calcarea Fluorica (Calc fluor, Fluor Spar, Fluoride of Lime).

Ulceration of mouth and throat, necrosis, pains, hard glands, cataract.

Mind: Depressed.

Head: Ulcerous scalp.

Eyes: Cysts, corneal spots, abscesses, conjunctivitis, cataract.

Ears: Deafness, suppuration.

Nose: Stinking green lumpy discharge, stuffiness, rhinitis.

Face: Swellings on jawbone.

Mouth: Gumboils, cracked tongue, loose teeth, pain chewing.

Throat: Pain, burning.

Stomach: Vomitting, flatulence, hiccough, indigestion.

Stool: Itches, cracks, bleeding, worms, haemorrhoids, gas.

Respiratory: Coughing, croup.

Circulation system: Vascular tumours, enlarged veins, valve diseases, heart, blood-vessel disease.

Neck: Lumbago, struggles to move.

Extremities: Pain and enlargement.

Skin: Cracks, fissures, callouses, ulcers, yellow pus, knots, swellings in fascia and tendons.

Calendula Officinalis (Calen, Marigold leaves and flowers).

Heals all wounds even long established ones, catarrh, certain deafness and helps with some cancers.

Head: Nervous, neck pains, scalp wounds.

Eyes: Suppuration of any small injuries.

Ears: Deaf, eczema, worse in damp.
Nose: Green discharge, one nostril running.
Stomach: Hunger, nausea, vomitting, distention.
Respiratory: Cough with green phlegm.
Skin: Abnormal, slough, yellowish, goose flesh.
Fever: Very cold.

Cannabis Indica (Can ind, Hashish).

Exaggerates sensations and emotions excessively, sooths mania, rages, nervous disorders.

Mind: Manic, uncontrolled, delirious, chronic vertigo.
Head: Shaking from side to side, pain with flatulence.
Eyes: Fixed expression.
Ears: Cannot take noise.
Face: Stupid expression, sticky dense saliva gumming lips together.
Stomach: Distended almost bursting, pain, appetite.
Urine: Thick mucus, oozes out.
Female: Sterile.
Respiratory: Struggles to breathe, asthma.
Heart: Palpitates, very slow beat.
Extremities: Heavy, paralytic, pains.

Cannabis Sativa (Can sat, Hemp).

Respiratory, urinary, sexual organs, exhaustion, choking, confusion.

Head: Vertigo, discomfort.
Eyes: Cataract, opaque, eyesight failing, aching eyeballs.
Respiratory: Struggle to breathe, rattles, green-bloody expectoration when coughing.
Heart: Irregular unusual beating.

Extremities: Heaviness, paralysis, problems under pads.
Worse: Lying down.

Cantharis (Canth, Spanish Fly).

Urinary and sexual organs, inflammation, gastro-intestinal disorder, lower bowel, haemorrhage, tries to urinate all the time, mucus secreted, bladder, kidneys, ovaries, meninges (brain, spine membrane), pleuritic (pleurisy) and pericardial (heart surrounds) inflammations.

Mind: Mania, howling, barking, delirium, rage, unconsciousness,

Head: Vertigo, disturbance.

Eyes: Fiery burning.

Face: Itches, burns.

Throat: Constricted, furred, red, burning, covered in vesicles, difficulty taking liquids, sticky discharge, laryngeal spasms if touched.

Chest: Hacking cough, blood, palpitation.

Stomach: Aversion to food and drink, vomit, pain, raging thirst.

Stool: Burning, dripping, bloody with shuddering.

Urine: Scalding and bloody, constant attempts to urinate, drops only.

Respiratory: Pleurisy, no voice power.

Heart: Palpitates, irregular, weak, pericarditis.

Extremities: Ulcers under pads, great limb pains, cannot walk.

Skin: Eczema, gangrene, eruptions, vesicular problems, burns, itches, inflammations, burning pads.

Worse: From touch or approach.

Better: From rubbing.

Carbo Vegetabilis (Carbo veg, Vegetable Charcoal).
Feeble circulation, no vitality, after disease, blue, decomposition, smelly.
Mind: Hates dark, memory poor.
Head: Itchy skin, vertigo, nausea.
Face: Mottled, puffy.
Eyes: Pain and vision problems.
Ears: Dry, peeling.
Nose: Tip red, scabby itching, bleeding, running, small eruptions, fluent coryza.
Mouth: Tongue white or yellow coated, gums soft and bleeding, teeth sore when chewing.
Stomach: Eructations, belching, pain, putrid and frightful smells, flatulence, nausea, distended abdomen, cramp.
Abdomen: Pain, colic, fetid flatus, huge abdomen, liver pain.
Rectum and stool: Itching, burning rectum, hot wet flatus, blood and oozing, bluish piles, cadaverous-smelling stool.
Respiratory: Coughing, gagging and mucus vomitting, wheezing and rattling, lung haemorrhage.
Extremities: Painful, weak, cramps, pain, almost paralysed.
Fever: Cold and thirsty.
Skin: Itchy, gangrenous, sores, bleeding, hairloss, ulcers, burning, stinking discharge, carbuncles, varicose ulcers.

Caroteus (Limited information).

Causticum (Caust, Tinctura acris sine Kali).
Rheumatism, arthritis, paralysis, deformities, tearing pains in muscle and fibre, catarrh, paralysis of vocal cords and tongue,

eyelids, bladder, extremities, warts, emaciation, constipation, urine retention.
Mind: Loving, sad.
Head: Frontal pains.
Face: Warts, jaw stiff, right side paralysed.
Eyes: Poor vision, staring eyes, cataract, ulcers on lids.
Ears: Catarrhal, blocked.
Nose: Ulcers and warts, ulcers, scaly, coryza.
Mouth: Bleeding gums, paralysis of tongue, lower jaw stiffness and pain.
Stool: Burning, piles, stool varies, often small, constipation.
Urine: Coughs and sneezes cause spurts, retention, very slow.
Respiratory: Swallowing, coughing, worse when warm, mucus, pains.
Extremities: Pains, single part paralysis, weakness, heaviness, shortened tendons, wobbly walk, falls, unsteady, rheumatism, stiffness, itches.
Skin: Bleeding warts, re-opening of old sores, problems in skin folds, sore behind ears.

❧

Chamomilla (Chamo, German Chamomile).
Emotion, irritability, restlessness, colic, no gumption, teething.
Mind: Moaning, sensitive, anger, irritation.
Head: Likely to hold at odd angle.
Ears: Pain, swelling, great discomfort.
Eyes: Jerking closed, lids not normal.
Nose: Pouring.
Face: Muscles and tongue twitch, aches, terrific discomfort.
Throat: Constricted and swollen.

Mouth: Salivates, especially at night.

Stomach: Yellow tongue, vomitting, eructations, terrible taste.

Abdomen: Flatulent distention, colic.

Stool: Haemorrhoids, pain, white and yellow colour, hot, slimy, fetid.

Respiratory: Raw throat, coughing, rattling, suffocating.

Back: Great pain, lumbago.

Extremities: Awful rheumatism, lower joints give way, paralysis at night.

Sleep: Eyes half open, moaning anxiety.

Chelidonium Majus (Chel, Celandine).

Liver, jaundice, lameness of single parts, lethargic, drainage remedy.

Head: Eyes streaming, vertigo, heavy and slow.

Eyes: Discoloured to yellowish, tiny pupils, tears.

Stomach: Yellow tongue with indentations, nausea, vomitting, pain, stench.

Abdomen: Distention, gallstones, liver and gall obstructed, enlarged liver.

Urine: Foamy, dark yellow, great quantities.

Stool: Round balls, can float, bright yellow, diarrhoea and constipation alternating, burning and itching anus.

Respiratory: Rapid puffing, coughs and rattles, lumps fly out of mouth, constricted breathing.

Neck: Stiff, sore, head pulled to the left.

Extremities: Pains, cannot be touched anywhere, rheumatism, partially paralysed.

Skin: Yellow itches, red spots, ulcers, cold and damp, bad smell.

China. Cinchona Officinalis (China, Peruvian Bark).

Loss of body fluids, exhaustion, prolonged fever.

Mind: Exhausted, debilitated.

Head: Frightful smashing pains, dizziness.

Eyes: Hollow eyes, distorted eyeballs, poor vision, sometimes nightblind.

Ears: Red and swollen, cannot touch.

Mouth: Tongue has dirty thick coat, teeth sore.

Stomach: Vomitting, does not eat, flatulence, indigestion, hiccough, belching and regurgitation.

Abdomen: Tight as a drum, colic, flatulence, liver and spleen enlarged, gallstones.

Stool: Yellow, frothy.

Male: Orchitis.

Respiratory: Difficulty breathing, suffocating, rattling, lung haemorrhage, asthma, has to hold head high and up.

Heart: Edema, anaemia, weak and strong beats.

Back: Severe pains.

Extremities: Pain which hard pressure eases, swollen joints, debility, weariness, trembling, cannot exert self.

Skin: Ulcers, caries, hot or cold in different places, very sensitive, dermatitis.

Sleep: Confused fear.

Fever: Intermittent, sneezes, weekly, chill, coryza.

Cholesterinum (Choles, Cholesterine from linings of inner ducts).

Liver cancer, gallstones, insomnia, pulmonary edema, cardiac pulsations, high blood pressure, yellow bags of cholesterol under lids and around eyes.

Cicuta Virosa (Cic, Water Hemlock, Fool's Parsley).

Nervous system, spasms, hiccough, tetanus, convulsions, bending head, neck and spine backwards, distortions, contortions, howling, skin disorder.

Mind: Delirium, playfulness, strange, epileptic.

Head: Meningitis, head twisted one side, fixed stare, convulsions, thick yellow crusts on skin, vertigo.

Eyes: Staring eyes cannot focus or gauge distance, pupils sometimes drawn up behind lids.

Ears: Bleeding, poor hearing.

Face: Yellow burning scabs and sores, pustules round mouth and nose, may grind teeth.

Throat: Dry, spasms, cannot swallow.

Stomach: Hiccough, thirst, eats strange things, frothing at mouth.

Abdomen: Colic, swollen, noisy, flatulent, painful to touch.

Rectum: Itches, must urinate with diarrhoea in morning.

Respiratory: Struggles to breathe.

Back and neck: Cramps, spasms, pulling head back spasmodically, back arched backward, cannot straighten bent limbs nor bend straight ones.

Skin: Yellow crusts, no itch, eruptions standing proud, suppression can lead to brain disease.

Cimicifuga Racemosa (Cim, Actaea Racemosa, Macrotys, Black Snake-root).

Brain, spine, muscles, female reproductive organs, cramps, pain anywhere, electric shocks, irritability.

Mind: Delirium, mania.

Eyes: Photophobia, eyeball pain.

Stomach: Nausea, vomitting, pointed and quivering tongue.

Respiratory: Coughing.

Heart: Weak pulse, stopping sometimes, suffocating.

Back: Spine cannot be touched, rheumatism.

Extremities: Twitching, aching, sore limbs, rheumatism, jerking, stiffness, heaviness.

Skin: Burning itches.

Cineraria (Cine, Dusty Miller).

Opaque eye, cataract, eye trauma.

External as well as internal use suggested, especially in case of trauma.

Cinnabaris – Mercurius Sulphuratus Ruber (Cinna, Mercuric Sulphide).

Head, skin, nose, ulceration, bones, pain, ulcers, buboes, nodes.

Eyes: Lids granulated, pain everywhere, redness.

Nose: Pain.

Throat: Dry with red ulcers in mouth and throat, stringy mucus discharge.

Male: Swelling, warts, chancres, buboes.

Extremities: Pain, especially when cold.

Clematis Erecta (Clem, Virgin's Bower).

Skin, glands, urinary system, genitals, emaciation, sleeplessness.

Cocaina (Coca, Cocaine, Erythroxylon Coca).
Anaesthetic, crawling itch, anxiety, headaches, breathlessness.

Coccidiosis Fowl (Coccid fowl).
Diarrhoea, shortened life span, 9 varieties affect chickens and 7 affect turkeys, remedy assists recovery or immunity. Pale, droopy, huddled, emaciated.

Coccus Cacti (Cocc cact, Cochineal).
Kidneys, bladder, catarrh of the bladder, spasmodic and whooping coughs.

Mind: Sad.

Head: Sore, scratches under eyelid.

Respiratory: Raw throat, coughing, suffocating, spasmodic coughs, bronchitis and mucus.

Heart: Pressure, discomfort.

Urine: Thick, dark, acidic, red sediment, constant desire to urinate.

Female: Clots in urine.

Coffea Cruda (Coff, Unroasted Coffee).
Nervous and vascular activity of all organs, agitation, excitability, uric acid, joint pains.

Mind: Excited, quick, irritable.

Head: Severe stabbing pains.

Mouth: Eats too fast, sore teeth.

Stomach: Great hunger.

Sleep: Moves, jumps, itches, sleepless.

Respiratory: Dry coughs.

Heart: Irregular rapid pulse.

Extremities: Pains, worse for moving and better for pressure.

Collinsonia Canadensis (Collin, Stone-Root).

Portal congestion, piles, constipation, catarrh of nasal, gastric and pharyngeal organs.

Head: Yellow-coated tongue catarrh.

Rectum: Dry, engorged haemorrhoids, pain, bleeding flatulence, constipation and diarrhoea alternating.

Female: Pain and swellings.

Respiratory: Dry hacking cough.

Heart: Edema, chest pains, palpitations, faintness.

Colocynthis (Coloc, Bitter Cucumber).

Cramp, twitching, pain, unbearable gut pains, irritability, shortening of muscles, contractions, abdomen and head, gall bladder, digestive spasms.

Mind: Irritable, angry.

Head: Vertigo, nausea, vomitting, sore skin, pain.

Eyes: Violent pains, especially in eyeballs.

Face: Swelling, pains, left side worse.

Stomach: Rough tongue, terrible hunger, pains.

Abdomen: Agonizing pains, colic, bruising, agitation, jelly stools odorous, distended.

Female: Internal tumours.

Urine: Discharge white and fetid, little crystals, burning, urine only expelled in small quantities.

Extremities: Muscles all contracted, cramped, pain, drawn together, stiffness, shortened tendons, joints sore.

Conium Maculata (Poison Hemlock in flower).

Ascending paralysis, suffocation, death. Wobbly gait, weakness, trembling, urinary troubles, debility, tumours, cancerous growths, glandular problems, impotence.

Mind: Timid, no interest, wants company but avoids company.

Head: Vertigo, averse to noise, nausea and vomitting from dizziness and pain.

Eyes: Averse to light, tears, corneal pustules, poor sight.

Ears: Bloody discharge, poor hearing.

Nose: Polyps, bleeding.

Stomach: Nausea, eructations, spasms, discomfort.

Abdomen: Swollen, bruised, cannot be touched.

Stool: Hard, burning, trembling after evacuation.

Urine: Retention, dribbles or flows and stops.

Male: Enlarged, stone-like testicles.

Respiration: Non-stop coughing, no breath, no air.

Extremities: Weak, quivering, paralysed.

Skin: Tumours, pains, ulcers, stinking discharges, burning skin.

⊷

Crotalis Horridis (Crot hor, Brazilian Rattlesnake venom).

Decomposing blood, unable to coagulate, haemorrhage, growths, fevers, sedated.

Mind: Rushed, depressed.

Head: Cannot run, jolting hurts head too much, vertigo, weakness and quivering.

Eyes: Yellowish, painful, photophobic, retinal haemorrhage.

Ears: Dizzy, blood escaping.

Nose: Black stringy discharge.

Face: Swollen lips, lockjaw.

Mouth: Smells mouldy, salivates, teeth grinding in sleep, tongue out to the right, bleeding tongue, cancer, bright red in centre.

Throat: Constricted, swollen, gangrenous, spasms, dark red, cannot swallow.

Stomach: Vomitting food and blood, dark green or black bile, cancerous stomach releasing slime and blood, ulcers, tightness, averse to meat, craves sweet things.

Abdomen: Hot, distended, swollen liver, cannot touch.

Stool: Black, thin, horribly offensive, bleeding, uncoagulated, oozing all the time.

Female: Pain.

Urine: Kidney swollen, bloody, dark urine.

Heart: Weakish, trembling, palpitating.

Respiratory: Bloody cough, tickling irritation.

Extremities: Trembling, swellings, right-sided paralysis.

Fever: Meningitis, Yellow-fever, haemorrhagic and putrid fevers.

Skin: Extreme pain, discolouration, yellowish, haemorrhaging, ulcers, suppuration, infection from the tiniest wounds, vaccinosis, septicaemia, lymphangitis, purple, mottled edemas, anthrax, boils, carbuncles, relieved by pressure.

Sleep: Yawning terribly, feels suffocated.

Cuprum Metallicum (Cup met, Copper).

Violent contractions, convulsions, cramps, spasmodic pain and attacks, epilepsy, nausea, foaming at mouth, falling, starts in left side. Tapeworm.

Head: Malicious, purple and red swellings with convulsions, giddiness, head falls forward.

Eyes: Fixed, crossed sometimes, rolling eyeballs.

Face: Contraction of jaws, foam.

Mouth: Tongue goes in and out, paralysis of tongue.

Stomach: Hiccough, nausea, vomitting, spasms, gurgling when drinking, colic, diarrhoea.

Abdomen: Hot, cannot touch, colic.

Stool: Black and bloody, pain.

Heart: Weak, failing, slow beat, palpitation, can be hard beat.

Respiratory: Coughing, suffocating, asthma.

Extremities: Cramps, coldness, weary, spasms, twitches and jerks.

Skin: Itching, ulcers, pimples in folds, psoriasis.

Sleep: Rumbling gut, loud.

ॐ

Digitalis (Digi, Foxglove).

Heart, weak, irregular beat, fibrillation, coldness, failing strength, blue, dying, breathless collapse.

Mind: Fearful, dull, slow pulse.

Head: Vertigo, pains, confusion, tongue and lips blue.

Eyes: Lids blue, margins red, swollen, agglutinated on waking, detached retina, poor vision.

Stomach: Nausea even after vomitting, weakness, worse for food, salivates, tender to touch.

Abdomen: Enlarged painful liver, severe pains all over.

Stool: White, like ash.

Urine: Wants to urinate all the time, burns, strong ammonia, thick, strangury, constriction.

Male: Edema of reproductive organs.

Respiratory: Cough, irregular breathing, tries to breathe deeply all the time, congestion, bloody sputum, cardiac edema.

Heart: Palpitates at any exertion, pulse too slow, heart failure.

Extremities: Swellings, coldness, rheumatic pains, weakness of muscles, enlarged joints.

Sleep: Jumps or starts as if falling.

Fever: Great heat and then weakness.

Skin: Edematous, red, spots, blue distended veins on eyes, nose and mouth, lips, tongue and ears, itches, worse on back.

Drosera (Dros, Sundew).

Kennel cough, whooping, coughs causing vomitting.

Head: Vertigo, can fall to the left.

Stomach: Nausea.

Respiratory: Spasmodic dry cough, hardly able to breathe, chokes, bleeding, retching, asthma.

Extremities: Pains and stiffness.

Dulcamara (Dulc, Bitter-Sweet).

Damp problems, skin eruptions, glands, stomach, mucus, rheumatism, spasms, paralysis of single parts.

Head: Confused, ringworm, crusts on head.

Nose: Blocked, yellow mucus, bloody crusts, coryza, tries to keep nose warm.

Eyes: Yellow discharge, hay fever.

Ears: Worry the animal, discomfort.

Face: Wet eruptions on skin.

Mouth: Salivates, stringy, tongue dry and rough, lip sores, face pains.

Stomach: Vomit white sticky mucus, thirst, cannot eat, nausea.

Abdomen: Colic, pains round umbilical area.

Stool: Mucus slimy green, bloody.

Urine: Thick with sediment, strangury, bladder catarrh when gets colds.

Respiratory: Coughing quantities of discharge, rattling, asthma.

Back: Stiff and lame.

Extremities: Warts, paralysis, icy cold, rheumatism, pain in the bones.

Skin: Itches and swellings, vesicular eruptions, boils, bleeding ulcers, humid eruptions, yellow crusts.

Fever: Dry, burning up.

Worse: At night, from cold.

Echinacea-Rudbeckia (Echin, Purple Cone-flower).

Septic condition, blood poisons, diarrhoea, boils, ulcers, gangrene, last stages of cancer to ease pain, poison bites or stings, meningitis, piles, suppuration, pus, disgusting discharge, debility.

Head: Dizziness, prostration.

Nose: Stinking, nauseating discharge, ulceration, post-nasal discharge, nose blocked, right nostril raw and bloody.

Mouth: Gums diseased, blood, mouth and lips cracked at edges, tongue brown, ulcerated and swollen, sometimes white coated with red edges, salivating.

Throat: Ulcerated, blackish.

Stomach: Belching, nausea.

Urine: No power, thick, involuntary.

Female: Offensive discharges.

Extremities: Aching limbs, weak, no energy.

Skin: Gangrenous ulcers, infection from small bites or wounds, boils, carbuncles.

Fever: Cold shivers.

Euphrasia (Euph, Eyebright).

Conjunctival membrane, lacrymation, nasal catarrh, offensive mucus.

Head: Pouring discharge from nose and eyes, pains, sight affected.

Nose: Pouring, coughing.

Eyes: Conjunctivitis, pouring tears.

Face: Top lip stiff.

Stomach: Vomit, nausea, hawking.

Rectum: Prolapse, dysentery, constipation

Male: Excrescences and growths, dribbling urine especially nights.

Respiratory: Yawning, throat full of discharge.

Skin: Red spots or pustules.

Ferrum Phosphoricum (Ferr phos, Phosphate of Iron).

Nervous, sensitive patient, no anxiety, chest troubles, bronchitis, tuberculosis, emaciation, wasting away, catarrh, anaemia, bright red bleeding from any orifice.

Head: Vertigo, painful to touch.

Eyes: Red, poor vision.

Ears: Poor hearing, infected, suppurations.

Nose: Colds, blood.

Face: Shakes head from side to side, hangs down.

Throat: Red, sore.

Stomach: Vomits undigested food and blood, averse milk and meat.

Abdomen: Haemorrhoids, dysentery, bloody discharge, undigested bloody watery stool.

Urine: Incontinent, spurts with cough.

Respiratory: Cough, blood, congestion.

Heart: Too fast, weak, cardiac disease.

Extremities: Stiff, pains, swellings, hot.

Sleep: Very bad.

Gelsemium (Gels, Yellow Jasmine).

Paralysis, dizziness, weak, slow, apathy, muscle groups can be paralysed, larynx, sphincters etc, sluggish, poor co-ordination.

Mind: Seeks solitariness.

Head: Vertigo, heavy eyelids, poor sight, sore skin, delirious.

Eyes: Can hardly open, almost or completely blind, cannot focus at all, inflammations, retinitis, detached retina.

Nose: Acute coryza.

Face: Quivering chin, dropped jaw.

Mouth: Yellow, coated, trembling tongue, stink, paralysis of tongue.

Throat: Raw, red, trouble swallowing.

Stomach: Hiccough, no thirst.

Stool: Paralysed rectum, involuntary stool, diarrhoea, possibly greenish.

Female: Infections.

Male: Burning itch and discharge,

Respiratory: Cannot breathe properly, collapse, cough, voice may vanish.

Heart: Too slow and weak.

Extremities: No control, cramps, weakness, fatigue.

Sleep: Unable to sleep properly.

Fever: Shaking, prostrate, chill, thirstless.
Skin: Itching eruptions, livid spots with stupor.

Glonoine   (Glon,   Gl=Glycerine/O=Oxygen/ N=Nitrogen, Nitro-glycerine).
Nerve disturbance, lassitude, irregularity of heart, itches, convulsions, pulsating pains, cerebral congestion, extremely high blood pressure.
Head: Dizzy confusion.
Eyes: Poor vision.
Mouth: Teeth painful.
Throat: Swollen under ears, choking.
Stomach: Nausea and vomitting, starving.
Abdomen: Constipation, itches, diarrhoea, piles, black lumpy stool.
Heart: Palpitations.

Golondrina (Golon, Euphorbia Polycarpa).
Immunity to snake poison or treatment of snake-bite.

Graphites (Graph, Black Lead, Plumbago).
Skin, constipation, anaemia, obesity, stomach ulcers, cancer of pylorus (between stomach and bowel), weak resolve, eczema, warts.
Mind: Timid, jumpy.
Head: Nosebleed (coupled with distended flatulence), may vomit, pains in head, teeth and neck, fetid, itchy eruption on head, catalepsy (rigid posture).
Eyes: Red, swollen, dry eyelids, blepharitis, eczema of lids, averse to artificial light.

Ears: Eruptions behind ears, cracks in ears, poor hearing.

Nose: Sores in nostrils.

Face: Burning, stinging pimples and eczema.

Mouth: Stink, too much saliva, blisters on tongue.

Stomach: Averse to meat, nausea and vomitting after meals, bloat.

Abdomen: Tight, flatulent, noisy, fetid smells, diarrhoea brown liquid.

Stools: Constipation, utterly nauseating smells, diarrhoea, prolapse, itches, burns, mucus, fissures.

Urine: Thick, stinking, with sediment.

Female: Disgusting, stinking discharges, cracked painful nipples.

Male: Eruptions, herpes (viral blisters).

Respiratory: Cannot breathe, constriction, pain.

Extremities: Pains, weakness, stiffness, cracks, fissures.

Skin: Hard, dry with eruptions, pus, rawness in crevices, ulcers, suppuration all over, possible edema.

❧

Guaco (Mikania, Climbing Hemp Weed).

Nervous system, female organs, antidote to poisonous bites and stings, cholera, cancer, deafness, tongue will not function properly, diarrhoea, dysentery.

Throat: Constricted, tongue too heavy to move properly.

Urine: Cloudy, painful.

Back: Pain down spine.

Extremities: Painful, heavy, paralysis of lower extremities.

❧

Hamamelis Virginica (Ham, Witch-hazel).

Bruises, venous haemorrhages, weakened coating of veins, passive haemorrhages, excellent for open wounds and blood loss or after surgery.

Eyes: Inflamed, bloodshot, weak.
Nose: Bleeding, bad smell from.
Throat: Red and blue.
Stomach: Thirst and discomfort.
Rectum: Raw and sore, bleeding piles, diarrhoea.
Urine: Bloody.
Female: Itches, pain.
Male: Orchitis.
Respiratory: Cough, some difficulty breathing.
Back: Severe pain, down into legs.
Extremities: Tired, painful muscles and joints.
Skin: Severe inflammations, ulcers, hotspots.

Hekla Lava (Hekla, Lava from Mt Hec(k)la).

Jaws, gum abscess, caries of bone, tumours, bone necrosis.

Face: Nasal bone ulcers, carious teeth, gum abscesses, sore teeth.

Hepar Sulphuris Calcareum (Hep sul(ph), Hepar Sulph, Calcium Sulphide).

Skin eruptions, swollen glands, boils, infections, abscesses, respiratory mucous membrane, catarrh, secretions, pus in nose, suppuration, stabbing pains, stimulates immune system.

Mind: Depressed and irritable.
Head: Vertigo, burning scalp itch.
Eyes: Corneal ulcers, iritis (iris inflamed), conjunctivitis, discharge, eyes and lids inflamed red, vision unclear, pains, may shake head.

Ears: Stinking pus, hearing poor, eczema.
Nose: Cheesy smell, discharge, sneezing, catarrh.
Face: Ulcers on mouth, pains everywhere.
Mouth: Gums and mouth bleeding.
Throat: Cannot swallow properly, chokes and gags.
Stomach: Distended, eructations.
Abdomen: Distended, pains.
Stool: Soft, yellow, fetid, muscles too weak to eject.
Urine: Drips and dribbles out, bladder weakened.
Male: Itches, warts, ulcers, bleeding.
Female: Old cheese smell, itches.
Respiratory: Awful cough, suffocating, wheezing, head back, anxiety, palpitations.
Skin: Suppurating, abscesses, cracks, ulcers, burning, stinging, cannot be touched, whole body smells bad.

∾

Histamine Hydrochloricum (Hist).
Allergies, eczema, allergies, rhinitis, strengthens immune system.
Nose: Itching, watering, running, sneezing, blocked ears.
Action: Inhibits histamine metabolism by signalling body that enough histamine has been made, and switches off further production and release.
Complementary remedies: Better when taken with **Kali Iodatum** for inflammation, and with **Succinic Acid** for exhaustion.

∾

Hydrophobinum (Hydroph, Lyssin, Saliva of Rabid Dog).
Nervous system, bone ache, convulsions after running water or flashing light.

Head: Acute senses.

Mouth: Spitting thick saliva, frothing, trying constantly to swallow, chokes when trying to drink water though has a raging thirst.

Respiratory: Chest spasms, may hold breath.

Stool: Sight or sound of water causes desire to empty bowels and bladder, watery stool. Constant attempts to urinate when near water or when in dazzling light.

Hyoscyamus (Hyos, Henbane).

Nervous system profoundly disturbed, mania, quarrelsomeness, agitation, weakness and twitching, spasms, delirium, toxic gastritis.

Mind: Foolish, crazy behaviour.

Head: Shaking back and forth, can lose consciousness.

Eyes: Wide-eyed, fixed gaze, harsh blinking.

Mouth: Tongue stuck, cracked, red, dry, foamy mouth, jaw hanging.

Throat: Constricted, unable to take in liquid.

Stomach: Convulsions, vomitting, hiccoughs, cramps, tenderness to touch.

Abdomen: Tight as a drum, painful, vomitting, belching, hiccoughing, colic.

Stool: Involuntary defecation, diarrhoea.

Urine: Un-noticed dribbling, bladder paralysed, no desire to urinate.

Chest: Suffocates, spasmodic cough, cannot lie down.

Sleep: Cannot sleep, has convulsions.

Extremities: Epilepsy, spasms, convulsions, cramps. Twitches non-stop.

Hypericum (Hyp, St John's Wort).
Nerve injuries, crushed limbs, excessive pain, prevents tetanus, after surgery, spasms, haemorrhoids, asthma, bites, puncture wounds.

Mind: Feels down.

Head: Pains all over and inside.

Stomach: Nausea, thirst, tongue white coated on inner half.

Rectum: Bleeding piles.

Extremities: Jerking and twitching, cramps, pains, bruising, tetanus.

Ignatia (Ign, St Ignatius's Bean).
Loss of co-ordination, too excitable, contradictory symptoms, rigid, trembling, hiccoughs, hysterical vomitting.

Mind: Brooding, changeable.

Head: Great pain.

Eyes: Lid spasms and pains.

Face: Constant twitches.

Mouth: Too much saliva, sore teeth.

Throat: Tries to swallow lump constantly, choking, inflammation and ulcers.

Stomach: Hiccoughs, bloat, cramps.

Abdomen: Rumbling colic.

Rectum: Itching, prolapse, haemorrhoids, constriction, diarrhoea, haemorrhage.

Respiratory: Hollow rapid coughs.

Extremities: Jerks and pain. Jerks in sleep.

Skin: Very itchy.

Indigo (Dye).

Epilepsy, grief, excitement, antidote for snake and spider poison.

Head: Convulsions, vertigo, nausea.

Nose: Sneezing and bleeding.

Stomach: Bloat, eructations.

Rectum: Weak, terrible itch.

Urine: Needs to urinate constantly, thick, mucus-filled, catarrhal.

Extremities: Pains, joint pain.

Nerves: Epilepsy, irritation.

Iodum (Iodine).

Wastes away but eats well, thin, weak, atrophy of all glands, tremor, inflammations, arthritis, connective tissue affected, edema, haemorrhage, catarrh, starvation.

Mind: Sudden escape or violence.

Eyes: Never steady, looking all over, red, running.

Nose: Great sneezing, running, blockage, ulceration.

Throat: Swollen glands, deafish, constriction.

Mouth: Bleeding soft gums, thickly coated tongue, disgusting ulcers and smells.

Stomach: Raging hunger and thirst with overproduction of gas, eats well.

Abdomen: Enlarged liver and spleen, pancreas problems.

Stool: Always accompanied by blood, frothy diarrhoea alternating with constipation.

Urine: Thick, dark yellow/green, huge amounts.

Male: Orchitis and atrophy.

Female: Haemorrhages.

Respiratory: Gasping cough, bloodspots, heart pumping wildly, wheezing, struggle to breathe.

Heart: Palpitations.
Extremities: Joint pains, swelling, rheumatism.
Skin: Yellow, aged, nodules.
Fever: Hot flushes.
Worse: When resting.

Ipecacuanha (Ipec, Ipecac-root).
Nausea, vomitting, spasmodic problems, bright red haemorrhages.
Mind: Irritation.
Head: Sore teeth and tongue.
Eyes: Red, dim, painful, burning eyelids.
Nose: Pouring but blocked, nausea.
Stomach: Clean tongue, vomitting of saliva and mucus with blood, salivates, face twitches.
Abdomen: Dysentery, pain, nausea, rigid body.
Stool: Green, frothy, slimy.
Female: Bright red bleeding.
Respiratory: Cannot breathe, sneezes and wheezes, coughs, bubbles and rattles, suffocating.
Sleep: Eyes half closed, jerks.
Extremities: Sudden jerks.

Jaborandi (Jabor, Pilocarpis Microphyllus).
Glandular stimulant, nausea, salivation, hot, secretions from all over can be copious, tremors.
Eyes: Weak, do not react, staring fixedly, tired, twitch.
Ears: Blocked up.
Mouth: Slimy saliva, too much saliva.
Stomach: Nausea and vomitting.
Abdomen: Diarrhoea.

Urine: Struggle to urinate.
Heart: Nervous, irregular, can collapse.
Respiratory: Raw throat, difficulty breathing, froth from edematous lungs.
Skin: Dry, itchy, eczema.

Kali Bichromicum (Kali bich, Bichromate of Potash).

All mucous membranes, catarrhs stringy and tough in pharynx, larynx, bronchii and nose, polyps, rheumatic and gastric symptoms alternate, perforated septum, affected are stomach, bowels, air passages, bones, fibrous tissue, kidneys, heart and liver, anaemia, weakness, cirrhosis, nephritis.

Head: Pains, disturbed vision.
Eyes: Swollen lids with stringy discharge, ulcers, conjunctivitis, iritis, inflammation.
Ears: Pain with yellow, stinking discharge.
Nose: Ulcerated septum (membrane between cavities), bad smell, thick stringy greenish discharge, sneezing with watery discharge, cannot breathe through nose.
Mouth: Shiny smooth dry tongue with dysentery, otherwise widened, flat with thick coating and indentations.
Throat: Raw, stringy discharge.
Stomach: Vomitting yellow, tight as a drum, ulcers, difficulty eating or drinking water, nausea.
Abdomen: Intestinal ulcers, pains.
Stool: Like jelly, some frothy dysentery alternating with plugged constipation.
Urine: Clogged with mucus, thick, pus, blood, cannot empty.
Male: Ulcers, itches, pustules.

Female: Prolapse, itch.

Respiratory: Cough, sticky expectoration, long sticky strings.

Extremities: Moving pains, bone pain, rheumatism, pain walking.

Skin: Eruptions and ulcers, pimples, itches.

৵

Kali Muriaticum (Kali mur, Chloride of Potassium).

Catarrhal infections, glandular troubles, grey tongue.

Head: Crusts, flakes.

Eyes: Scabs, pus, ulcers, opacity.

Ears: Infections and swellings, discharge.

Nose: Thick catarrh, white, bleeding, blockage.

Face: Swollen cheeks.

Mouth: Ulcers, tongue grimy, slimy grey-white, swollen neck glands.

Stomach: Mucus, vomitting, water assuages hunger, salivation, constipation.

Abdomen: Swollen, tender, bloat, thread-worms, itchy anus.

Stool: Dark bleeding piles, thick blood, changing light-coloured stools with constipation, to diarrhoea with clay-coloured stools.

Respiratory: Constant loud coughing, rattling, voiceless, suffering.

Extremities: Painful, swollen joints, rheumatic pains, stiffness.

Skin: Pus-filled pimples, scales, eczema, swollen bursae (sacs).

৵

Kali Phosphoricum (Kali phos, Phosphate of Potassium).

Collapse, moveless, no nerve power, depression, decay, gangrene, malignant tumour, after removal of cancer. For physical and psychological weakness.

Mind: Anxiety, irritation, brain fag, hysteria, terrors.

Head: Vertigo, exhaustion, ache.

Eyes: Half closed, poor sight. Hollow eyed.

Nose: Nauseating discharge and smell.

Mouth: Tongue brown coated, sore teeth, bleeding gums receding, red strip in gums, fetid breath.

Throat: Gangrenous, voiceless.

Stomach: Sick feeling constantly.

Abdomen: Foul diarrhoea, especially while eating, blood, swollen tight, prolapse.

Urine: Too yellow, incontinent, bleeding.

Respiratory: Breathless, worse after food, asthma.

Extremities: Lame, paralysed, pain.

Kali Sulphuricum (Kali sulph, Potassium Sulphate).

Awful yellow mucus discharges, inconstant, copious.

Head: Scurf, bald spots.

Ears: Pus discharge, poor hearing.

Nose: Swollen inflamed inside, breathes through mouth.

Stomach: Nausea, vomitting, thirst, sore gums, yellow-coated slimy tongue.

Abdomen: Haemorrhoids, constipation, slimy yellow diarrhoea, colic, cannot be touched, tight as a drum.

Male: Orchitis, discharges.

Respiratory: Cough, rattle, asthma.

Extremities: Pains travelling all over.
Skin: Burns, itches, polyps, rash, ringworm, scales.

Kreosotum (Kreos, Beechwood Kreosote).

Gangrene, puffiness, haemorrhage, ulcers, cancers, burning and stinking discharges, pulsations, bleeding from any small injury, rotten teeth from babyhood, foul smell.

Mind: Stupid, irritable.
Eyes: Red, swollen.
Ears: Poor hearing, skin eruptions.
Mouth: Teeth rotten and loose, gums spongy, bleeding, red lips bloody, putrid smell.
Nose: Constant discharge and bad odour, catarrh.
Throat: Choking all the time, stench.
Stomach: Vomitting, nausea.
Abdomen: Green stinking stool with blood, offensive dark diarrhoea, burning piles, painful distention.
Urine: Itching, retention, stinking, wets sleeping place.
Female: Violent itching, discharges, bleeding, stink, pain.
Respiratory: Cough, gangrenous lungs, tries to vomit.
Back: Weak, no strength.
Extremities: Joint pain.
Skin: Itching, burning, gangrene, bleeding, eruptions and infections, herpes, eczema.
Sleep: Very disturbed.

Lachesis (Lach, Bushmaster Snake, Surucucu).

Haemorrhage, decomposition of blood, septic infections, poisonings, prostration, delirium.

Mind: Jealous, restless, suspicious.

Head: Vertigo, avoids the sun.

Eyes: Weak vision.

Nose: Sneezing, bleeding, short of breath.

Face: Swollen.

Mouth: Swollen, red, dry tongue, nausea, pain.

Throat: Raw, septic, black/blue, starts on left side, trying to swallow all the time makes it worse.

Stomach: Painful to touch, pressure, hunger, trembling, painful swallowing.

Abdomen: Like a drum.

Stool: Prolapse, haemorrhage, constipation, odorous stool.

Lacticum Acidum (Lact ac, Lactic Acid).

Rheumatism, ulceration of vocal cords.

Stomach: Raging hunger, nausea, mucus.

Throat: Keeps swallowing, salivates.

Extremities: Rheumatism, pain, weakness, trembling.

Lathyrus Sativa (Lath sat, Chick-pea).

Yawning, poor recovery from illness, no nerve power, Beri-beri in humans, spasticism followed by paralysis in lower extremities.

Mind: Depressed, no interest.

Extremities: Wobbly, rigid, spastic gait, cramps, paralysis, emaciated, blue, stiff, lame.

Ledum (Led, Marsh-Tea).

Rheumatism from bottom up, skin eruptions, cold but averse to heat, good for puncture wounds and bites, use for Tetanus especially with twitching muscles near wound, good for insect bites.

Head: Nosebleed, vertigo.

Eyes: Cataracts, pains.

Face: Possible spots, discharge around nose and mouth.

Respiratory: Coughing bloody mucus, short of breath, spasmodic coughs.

Rectum: Haemorrhoids and fissures.

Extremities: Hot, swollen, pain, easily sprained.

Skin: Terribly itchy feet and ankle, eczema on body.

Lilium Tigrinum (Lil tig, Tiger-lily).

Ovaries, uterus, heart, small spots of pain, rheumatic arthritis.

Mind: No interest.

Eyes: Pain, impaired vision, tears.

Stomach: Flatulent, craves meat, raging thirst.

Abdomen: Tight, painful.

Urine: Milky, hot, constant desire to urinate.

Stool: Constant pressure in rectum.

Heart: Palpitation, irregular pulse, too quick.

Extremities: Unsteady, aches pains, burning feet.

Lobelia Inflata (Lob, Indian Tobacco).

Pneumo-gastric nerve, poor respiration, nausea, vomitting.

Head: Prostration, fear, vertigo.

Ears: Discharges, eczema, deafness.

Mouth: Salivates, sticky mucus on white-coated tongue.

Stomach: Flatulent, breathless, nausea, vomitting, salivating, burning.

Respiratory: Cannot breathe, emphysema, cough, constriction.

Back: Cannot be touched at all.

Urine: Dark, thick, red, heavy sediment.
Skin: Awful prickling with great nausea.

Lycopodium (Lyco, Club Moss spores).
Urinary and digestive, liver function, kidneys, bloody urine, emaciation, weakness, withered, no power in Vital Force.
Mind: Fearful, timid.
Head: Shaking, twisting mouth, vertigo, hair falling out, eczema.
Ears: Revolting discharge, eczema, poor and disturbed hearing.
Nose: Blocked, running, back of throat discharge, crusts.
Face: Itches, lower jaw hangs open, shrunken look.
Mouth: Salivates, tongue blisters, stench, black cracked tongue, herpes.
Throat: Vomits through nose, raw, red, tongue moves to and fro, ulcers.
Stomach: Starving, bloated, hiccough.
Abdomen: Drum-like, dropsy, hernia, liver disorder.
Stool: Diarrhoea, constipation, haemorrhoids, pain.
Urine: Retention, pains, red sediment.
Respiratory: Coughing, burning, bloody expectorations, catarrh, pneumonia.
Heart: Diseased, palpitates.
Back: Burning pains.
Extremities: Pain, heaviness, sore under pads, cramps, twitches and jerks.
Skin: Abscessed, itchy, violent irritation, spots and growths, stinking, dropsy.

Lyssin (see Hydrophobinum).

Magnesia Phosphorica (Phosphate of Magnesia).
Anti-spasmodic, the homeopathic aspirin, cramp, pain, neuralgia.
Mind: Full of the pain.
Head: Vertigo on moving.
Eyes: Hot, twitchy, blurred, tears, worse on right side.
Ears: Pains.
Mouth: Swollen tongue, toothache, ulcers, swollen face glands.
Throat: Puffy, painful, stiff.
Stomach: Hiccoughs, retching.
Abdomen: Pressure, flatulence, pain, sensitivity, belching, flatus constantly released, constipation.
Respiratory: Raw larynx, asthma, spasmodic cough.
Heart: Palpitation.
Extremities: Cramps, quivering, twitching, pains, general weakness.

Mercurius Corrosivus (Merc cor, Corrosive Sublimate).
Rectum, bladder, destroys secreting part of kidneys, slow action, ulcers in gut, bleeding diarrhoea, mucus and blood in urine, ulceration in mucus membranes.
Nose: Mucus membrane, dry, red pouring bloody.
Eyes: Ulceration of eyelids.
Ears: Nauseating pus.
Face: Lips black and swollen.
Mouth: Loose teeth, purple infected gums, salivation.
Throat: Raw, cannot swallow properly.

Stomach: Green vomit, unceasing.
Abdomen: Bloated, painful.
Stool: Hot bloody slimy, stinking.
Respiratory: Coughing bloody mucus.
Urine: Green, thick with blood, hot.
Male: Orchitis.

Mercurius Hydrargyrum (Merc hyd, Quicksilver).
See Mercurius Solubilis Hahnemanni.

Mercurius Solubilis Hahnemanni (Merc sol, Mercury, Quicksilver).
Blood, mucus membranes, salivary glands, liver, kidneys, bones and joints, mouth problems, glands, conjunctivitis.
Mind: Willpower gone, no interest in life.
Head: Fetid eruptions on scalp, hair loss, oily head.
Eye: Red thick swollen lids, iritis.
Ears: Stinking bloody yellow discharge, boils.
Nose: Sneezing, yellow green stinking discharge, thick, hanging, bleeds.
Mouth: Jelly-like gums, bleeding, decayed teeth which are loose, tongue yellow flabby with furrow down middle and ulcers, nauseating fetid smell near patient.
Throat: Constantly swallowing, ulcers.
Stomach: Feels full and tight, hiccoughs, putrid regurgitation.
Abdomen: Flatulent distention, stool green bloody slimy, occasionally white grey.
Urine: Green, bloody, thick.
Respiratory: Paroxysms of coughs with catarrh.
Extremities: Bone pain, swelling of feet and legs.

Skin: Moist, eruptions, ulcers, pimples, crusts, suppuration, buboes, orchitis.

Mercurius Vivus (Merc viv, Quicksilver, Mercury).
Digestive tract, kidney failure, chicken-pox, colds with pain in nose, diarrhoea, mouth ulcers, earache with discharge, influenza, over-salivation, infectious diseases, suppurative conditions.

Nose: Pours.

Rectum: Painful diarrhoea.

Ears: Pus discharge.

Eyes: Red and irritated.

Mouth: Ulcerous with burning raw throat, toothache, salivation.

Millefolium (Mille, Yarrow).
Bright red haemorrhages, hernia, pox, after fall from height, overstraining, temperature too high for too long.

Head: Epilepsy, convulsions, vertigo.

Snout (nose): Bleeds.

Stool: Bleeding piles.

Urine: Bloody.

Female: Bright red haemorrhages.

Respiratory: Coughs blood, palpitations.

Muriaticum Acidum (Mur ac, Muriatic Acid from Hydrochloric Acid).
Septic blood conditions, fever, prostration, high temperature, decomposition of fluids, bowel evacuates involuntarily while urinating, haemorrhages, mouth and anus.

Mind: Sad, peevish.

Head: Vertigo.

Nose: Sneezing, bleeding.

Face: Jaw hangs down, dry, cracked lips.

Mouth: Swollen dry hard tongue with bumps deep ulcers and terrible smell, gums infected.

Throat: Raw, ulcerous, swallowing causes choking.

Stomach: Ravenously hungry and thirsty, averse to meat.

Rectum: Haemorrhoids, itches, prolapse, terribly sensitive to touch, bowel empties while urinating.

Heart: Weak and irregular.

Female: Ulcers in genitals.

Extremities: Tottering, painful.

Skin: Stinking ulcers, growths, eruptions, itches, eczema.

Naphthaline (Naphth, from Coal-tar, Tar Camphor).

Cough, urinary organs irritation, hay fever, coryza.

Head: Stupefied.

Eyes: Detached retina, deposits upon retina, cataract, opacity of cornea.

Urine: Urgent need to urinate, black urine, awful smell of decomposing

Natrum Muriaticum (Nat mur, Chloride of Sodium).

Salt retention, dropsies and edemas, blood changes resulting in anaemia, tissue changes giving gouty symptoms; intermittent fevers; problems with alimentary tract and skin; debility, weakness, emaciation, weightless from digestive problems.

Mind: Depressed, irritable, avoids company.

Head: Pain, sore eyes.

Eyes: Drooping, burning, pus, tears, swollen lids, cataract threatening.

Ears: Bothersome noises in ears.

Nose: Fluent coryza three days then complete blockage, violent sneezing.

Mouth: Bubbles on tongue and in mouth, feeling as if hair was stuck on it, eruptions on lips, ulcers and cracks, lower lip cracked.

Stomach: Raging thirst, hunger, abdomens distended tightly, cough.

Rectum: Burning, itching, bleeding, constipation, diarrhoea.

Urine: Sometimes involuntary passing, but very slow when urinating.

Female: Prolapses.

Respiratory: Coughs with spurts of urine, short of breath.

Heart: Palpitating, fluttering.

Extremities: Weak, twist sometimes.

Sleep: Jerking, sleepless.

Skin: Eruptions, blisters, itch, burn, grease, crusts, eczema, hives.

Good for convalescence.

Nitricum Acidum (Nit ac, Nitric Acid).

Action on ports where mucus membrane and skin meet; blisters and ulcers – mouth tongue and genitals, bleeding, fissures in rectum, all discharges disgusting, diarrhoea, arthritis.

Mind: Ugly, malicious, nasty.

Head: Hair falls out, sensitive skin.

Ears: Poor hearing.

Eyes: Iritis, tears, photophobia, ulceration.

Nose: Bleeding, stinking catarrh, running, coryza, red tip, green or yellow mucus.

Mouth: Tongue red and clean, groove in middle with pimples, loose teeth, spongy bleeding gums, fetid breath, salivating.

Throat: Dry, cough.

Abdomen: Constipation, cracked rectum, prolapse, violent pain, bleeding, haemorrhoids, sometimes slimy and offensive diarrhoea.

Urine: Stinks, bloody, thick and mucus-filled.

Male: Ulcers, offensive discharge.

Female: Ulcers, hairless sometimes, discharges externally.

Respiratory: Breathless, coughing.

Skin: Ulcers, rawness, warts (bleeding sometimes).

Nux Vomica (Nux v, Poison-nut).

For quick, nervous irritable patients, digestive disturbances, portal problems, convulsions, fiery attitude, out of step, spasmodic.

Mind: Sullen, irritable, cannot take noise, light.

Head: Pain, vertigo, giddiness.

Eyes: Atrophy of optic nerve, photophobia.

Ears: Itch deep inside, pain with noise.

Nose: Blocked, running, bleeding.

Mouth: Swollen white gums, bloody saliva, ulcers, back of tongue has deep fur, front clean, gums bloody.

Stomach: Ravenous, nauseous, vomitting, retching, bloat.

Abdomen: Distention pressing gut out of place, flatulence, painfully engorged liver.

Stool: Constipation, ineffectual desire to expel, itching haemorrhoids.

Urine: Small quantities frequently. Strangury.

Male: Orchitis.

Female: Prolapse.

Respiratory: Cough, asthma, constriction, panting, some blood.

Extremities: Loss of power.

Skin: Red itches, blotches, urticaria.

Onosmodium (Onos, False Gromwell).

Concentration and co-ordination disturbed, vertigo, prostration, tiredness, frigidity.

Mind: Confused.

Eyes: Weak.

Throat: Raw, dry.

Abdomen: Distention, great thirst.

Chest: Pain, irregular pulse.

Female: Discharge, pain.

Extremities: Unsteady, weak, wobbly, tired.

Opium (Papaver Somniferum, Dried Latex of Poppy).

Stupor, torpor, painless, stupid.

Mind: No contact with the world.

Head: Brain paralysis, delirius, vertigo.

Eyes: Half closed, no dilation or reaction.

Face: Twitching, distorting.

Mouth: Black paralysed tongue, blood froth, difficult to swallow.

Stomach: Convulsions and vomitting.

Abdomen: Drum-like, rock hard faeces.

Rectum: Severe pain, constipation, spasmodic stooling black and frothy, odorous.

Urine: No pressure, weak stream.

Female: Threatened abortion, terrible pains.

Respiratory: Breathing stops on sleeping must be shaken to re-start, difficulty breathing, cough, bloody sputum.

Sleep: Goes into coma.

Extremities: Paralysis, twitching, convulsions, jerking.

Passiflora Incarnata (Pass, Passion Flower).

Anti-spasmodic, coughs, delirium tremens, disturbed cerebral functions, Tetanus, hysteria, sleeplessness, flatulence with eructations, convulsions.

Petroleum (Petro, Crude Rock-oil).

Catarrh, mucus, gastric problems, skin disorders.

Mind: Irritable, confused.

Head: Wet skin eruptions, vertigo.

Eyes: Poor sight, fissures, scurfy skin, eyelashes fall out.

Ears: Itches, fissures, deafness, irritation, poor hearing, eczema.

Nose: Cracks, burning, ulcers, discharge.

Stomach: Distension, hunger after stool, nausea, ravenous.

Abdomen: Watery daytime diarrhoea.

Phosphorus (Phos).

Mucus membranes degenerating, irritated, inflamed; spine and nerves affected, paralysis, bone degeneration especially lower jaw and tibia; degeneration of blood vessels and every tissue and organ, haemorrhage, nervous debility, emaciation, sudden prostration, cirrhosis, caries; muscular hypertrophy (over-growth), scurvy, weak bones.

Mind: Up and down, over-sensitive, jumpy.

Head: Brain fag, itches on skin, vertigo.

Eyes: Poor sight, photophobia, pains, cataract, atrophy of optic nerve.

Ears: Poor hearing.

Face: Swelling of jaw, looks ill.

Mouth: Ulcerated gums, smooth clean red or white dry tongue, thirst.

Stomach: Vomitting and belching.

Stool: Fetid and difficult to expel when long and hard, exhausting green diarrhoea, involuntary discharge sometimes, blood, white stools sometimes, bleeding.

Urine: Brown with red sand.

Female: Offensive, watery discharge.

Respiratory: Hacking raw cough, tightness, pneumonia, bloody saliva.

Heart: Anxious rapid beating.

Extremities: Paralysis from bottom up, weakness, trembling, collapsing joints.

Sleep: Wakes all the time, unrefreshed.

Fever: Delirium, starving but no thirst.

Skin: Bleeding from smallest injury, cold, scurvy, ulcers, fungous infections.

Worse: Touch, heat, exertion.

Better: Dark, cold, open air, lying down.

Phosphoric Acidum (Phos ac, Phosphoric Acid).

Debility, exhaustion, flatulence, diarrhoea, haemorrhages, relieves pain of cancer, serious depression, bone disorders especially in the young.

Phytolacca (Phyto, Poke-root).
Prostration, aching, glands, fibrous and osseous tissue, fasciae and sheathes, scar tissue, rheumatism, bone-pain, thin, sore throat.

Mind: Cares about nothing.

Head: Rheumatism, pain, scaly scalp.

Eyes: Tearful, scratchy, burning.

Nose: Copious flow of water, especially one nostril and back of throat.

Mouth: Tetanic clench, lower lip down to expose teeth, head down, red-tipped tongue with yellow centre stripe, indented, blood and blisters in mouth, stringy saliva.

Throat: Dark and painful, swollen, thick sticky mucus, ulcers.

Abdomen: Pain, constipation, rectum bleeding.

Urine: Pain, suppressed, small quantities.

Female: Possible mammary abscesses and tumours.

Male: Great pains under pelvis.

Respiratory: Cannot breathe, hacking cough.

Back: Stiff, with pain.

Extremities: Shoulder pain, rheumatism, shifting pains, under thighs, under paws, swellings, sore legs.

Skin: Boils, itches, lesions, eruptions, buboes, warts, moles, growths.

Picric Acid (Pic ac, Trinitrophenol).
Degeneration of spinal cord, prostration, weakness, pain, debility, pernicious anaemia, spasms, shakes.

Mind: Will not do anything, demented.

Head: Boils in ears and neck, anxiety, brain fag.

Eyes: Conjunctivitis, thick yellow discharge.

Stomach: Cannot stand food.

Urine: Dark, bloody, small quantities every time, dribbling.

Extremities: Exhaustion, spine burning, cold, paralysis from the lowest points progressing upwards.

Pilocarpus Microphyllus (Jaborandi).

See Jaborandi.

Plumbum (Plum m, Lead).

Paralysis of forelegs or forearms, preceded by pain, blood; alimentary and nervous systems; red corpuscles diminish in number, anaemia, grey colour, deliriums, coma, convulsions; muscular atrophy, multiple sclerosis.

Mind: Depression, fear, apathy.

Head: Delirium.

Eyes: Yellow, inflamed, loss of sight possible.

Face: Shiny, greasy, deathly.

Mouth: Swollen bluish gums, tongue tip red, tongue almost paralysed.

Stomach: Tight as a drum, vomits, cannot eat solids.

Abdomen: Flatus, colic, pain.

Rectum: Black constipation, constricted.

Urine: One drop at a time.

Heart: Weak.

Skin: Yellow, spotted, dry.

Extremities: Paralysis, especially single parts, pains, cramp, twitching, swellings, atrophy.

Podophyllum (Podo, May-apple).

Duodenum, small intestines, liver and rectum, gastro-enteritis, vomitting, gushing profuse jelly-like mucus, very offensive from rectum, prolapsed uterus, torpid liver.

Mind: Delirium.

Head: Moves side to side, eyes half closed, vomitting, moaning.

Tongue: Too wide, foul.

Stomach: Vomitting, froth, gagging.

Abdomen: Tight, rumbling flatus.

Rectum: Green watery diarrhoea, prolapse, clay-coloured hard constipation, piles.

Female: Prolapse, haemorrhage.

Extremities: Pains, paralysis on left.

Psorinum (Psor, Scabies Vesicle).

Cold patients, debility, no reaction, filthy smelling secretions, major skin problems.

Mind: No motivation for anything.

Head: Great pain.

Eyes: Blepharitis, acid, red at edges.

Mouth: Ulcerated, mucus on palate.

Nose: Terrible catarrh, blocked, coryza.

Ears: Revolting discharge, awful itches, brown pus, oozing red around.

Face: Sickly, swollen top lip.

Throat: Difficulty swallowing.

Stomach: Starving.

Stool: Fetid, bloody, liquid.

Chest: Unable to breathe properly.

Extremities: Weak.

Skin: Dry, dirty, oily, itchy, ulcerated, eczema, crusts.

Pulsatilla (Puls, Wind Flower).
All mucous membranes, always appears unhappy, constantly changing.
Mind: Timid, emotional, no power.
Head: Vertigo, pains.
Ears: Swollen, stinking discharge, hearing impaired.
Eyes: Itching, burning, full of mucus, conjunctivitis.
Nose: Bad smell, green or yellow mucus, blocked, no smell.
Mouth: Swollen lower lip, dry, licks constantly, tongue mucus covered, stink, crack in lower lip, mucus covered yellow or white tongue, no taste.
Stomach: Eructations, flatulence, no thirst, vomitting, pain, hunger.
Abdomen: Colic, tight as a drum, rumbling.
Stool: Changes all the time, watery, bloody, two or three normal stools per day, haemorrhoids.
Urine: Dribbling, especially with sneeze or flatus.
Male: Orchitis, drops of urine only.
Respiratory: Coughing, pain, short of breath, anxiety, palpitation, smothered feeling.
Sleep: Afternoons must sleep, cannot sleep in evenings.
Back: Shooting pains between shoulders.
Extremities: Pain, moving constantly, swollen joints, sore pelvic joints, pain under pads inflamed.
Skin: Varicose veins, itches, urticaria.

Pyrogenium (Pyro, Artificial Sepsin).
Septic states, restless, typhoid, typhus, ptomaine poisoning,

diphtheria, infected wounds, miscarriage, awful smelling discharges, breath diarrhoea and vomit foul, violent pain and burning in abscesses, threatening heart failure.

Mind: Restless, disturbed.

Head: Throbbing.

Mouth: Tongue smooth, dry, red, shiny, nausea, stench of breath.

Stomach: Vomitting, drinks water then vomits when it warms.

Abdomen: Bladder and rectum piercing pain, distended gut.

Stool: Disgusting, inertia of bowel, black faeces.

Heart: Palpitation, tiredness.

Female: Sepsis, infection, frightful smell.

Fever: Cold.

Extremities: Aching pains, morning exhaustion.

Skin: Quick infection of the slightest injury.

Should only be used by a professional homeopath.

Ranunculus Bulbosus (Ranunc b, Buttercup).

Muscle tissue and skin, chest walls, hiccough, shooting pains.

Head: Irritability, pain in head and eyes.

Eyes: Photophobia, spots on cornea.

Chest: Pain, pain to touch, abdomen tender.

Skin: Itching, burning eruptions, chapping, blisters.

Rescue Remedy (Dr. Bach's Flower Remedies).

Shock, trauma, fear, confusion, terror, panic, apprehension, stress.

Rhododendron (Rhod, Snow-rose).

Rheumatism, worse before storms, pains all over, joints painful.

Mind: Terror of storms or thunder.

Head: Eye and head pains.

Ears: Hearing poor.

Mouth: Swollen gums, loose teeth.

Chest: Breathless, pain, stitches.

Male: Orchitis.

Extremities: Pain, stiffness, swollen joints, worse before or during weather changes.

Rhus Toxicodendron (Rhus t, Poison Ivy).

Skin, rheumatic pains, mucous membranes, fevers, joints, tendons, sheaths causing pain and stiffness, motion loosens patient, physical strain, septic conditions, septicaemia.

Mind: Fears.

Head: Pains, itchy skin.

Ears: Swollen, pus discharge.

Nose: Sneezing, ulcerated, swollen, bleeds.

Face: Jaw dislocates.

Mouth: Tongue red on tip and along sides, cracks, teeth loose, gums infected.

Throat: Struggles to swallow.

Stomach: No appetite, thirst, bloat after eating.

Abdomen: Pains, distention, rumbling.

Rectum: Diarrhoea, blood, slime.

Ruta Graveolens (Rue-bitterwort).

Periosteum, cartilages, eyes and uterus, tendons, pain, bruises, lameness, lassitude.

Head: Pain.
Stomach: Gastralgia, unhappy.
Urine: Keeps trying to urinate.
Rectum: Constipation alternating with mucus, blood, prolapse.
Respiratory: Breathless, coughing.
Back: Pain in mornings.
Extremities: Pain and stiffness everywhere.

Sabadilla (Sabad, Cevadilla seed, Asagraea Officialis).
Mucous membrane of nose, and lachrymal gland, hayfever-like symptoms, coryza, sensitive to cold, ascarides.
Head: Burning, red eyes, running tears.
Nose: Sneezing and running, copious discharge.
Throat: Constant swallowing.
Extremities: Cracks under toes and toe nails.
Skin: Thickened, deformed, itching anus.

Sabina (Savine, Juniperus Sabina new branches).
Miscarriages, haemorrhage, strong pulsations, needs fresh air.
Abdomen: Colic, distended like drum.
Rectum: Bleeding with bright red blood, constipation.
Urine: Bloody, retention, bladder inflamed and throbbing.
Female: Threatening miscarriages, haemorrhages.
Extremities: Shiny, swollen, red, arthritic joints.
Skin: Itching, burning, fig warts.

Secale Cornutum-Claviceps Purpurea (Sec, Ergot).

Contraction of certain muscle fibre; anaemia, gangrene, coldness, shrivelled skin, oozing haemorrhages, thin stinking black blood, emaciation, diminished pancreatic fluid, strong hunger and thirst, inflamed arteries.

Head: Drawn back, dark blood from nose.

Face: May distort.

Mouth: Dry cracked tongue with thick yellow coat, swollen and paralysed.

Stomach: Vomitting blood, stench.

Rectum: Wide open and involuntary green bloody stinking stools.

Urine: Black blood, retention, bladder paralysis.

Female: Threatened abortions.

Chest: Cramp, pain, palpitation.

Extremities: Staggering, pains.

Skin: Shrivelled, bluish, gangrenous, boils with green pus.

Fever: Cold.

❧

Sepia (Sep, Cuttlefish Juice).
Tendency to abortion, uterine problems.
Mind: Indifference to loved ones, irritable.
Head: Jerking head backwards and forwards.
Nose: Green discharge, chronic catarrh.
Ears: Swellings, eruptions, herpes.
Mouth: Tongue white, swollen cracked lower lip.
Abdomen: Great discomfort, bloat.
Rectum: Bleeding, large hard stools, prolapse.
Urine: Red with sand in it.
Respiratory: Cough, cannot breathe properly.
Heart: Violent palpitations – sometimes.
Extremities: Lame and stiff.

Fever: Flushes of heat, but cold, damp.
Skin: Itches, ringworm, urticaria, odour.

Silicea (Sil, Silica, Flint).

Poor digestion, bad nutrition, disease of bone, necrosis, fibrotic, deep and slow action abscesses, epilepsy, slow gait, cold patient, no vital heat, body and mind debilitated, pus formations, no fortitude, recurrent infections, effects of vaccinations.

Mind: Faint-hearted.

Eyes: Aversion to light, cataract, abscess after injury, opacity.

Ears: Stinking discharge.

Nose: Crusts and terrible itches, perforation of septum.

Mouth: Boils on gums, abscesses under teeth.

Stomach: Excessive thirst, vomits after drinking.

Abdomen: Swollen hard, grumbling.

Rectum: Paralysed, cracks, bad smell.

Urine: Bloody with sediment, involuntary discharge.

Male: Thick fetid discharge.

Female: Itches, ulcers, abscesses, cysts, lumps.

Respiratory: Unable to shake off effects of snuffles and chills, violent coughing.

Extremities: Cramps, pains, paralysis.

Skin: Ulcers, cracks, blotches, boils, abscesses, stinking pus.

Sinapsis Nigra, Brassica Nigra (Syn nig, Black Mustard).

Lumpy secretions from nose, hayfever, coryza, pharyngitis, pox.

Head: Hot itches.

Nose: Dry, blocked, sneezing, running.
Throat: Wheezing, great coughing spells.
Stomach: Breath stinking, mouth full of cankers.
Urine: Copious.
Back: Pain, keeps patient awake.

Spigelia (Spig, Pinkroot).
Heart, eye and nervous system, neuralgia, anaemia, debilitation, rheumatism, scrofulous, pains, symptoms of worms.
Head: Vertigo and pain.
Eyes: Severe pain in sockets.
Nose: Chronic discharge.
Mouth: Offensive smell, fissured painful tongue.
Heart: Violent palpitation, weak pulse.
Rectum: Crawling itches, ascarides.
Worse: For touch, motion.

Spongia Tosta (Spong, Roasted Sponge).
Respiratory organs, heart, swollen glands, exhaustion, difficulty breathing, no voice.
Mind: Anxiety.
Eyes: Gummed up.
Nose: Running, alternating with blockage.
Mouth: Tongue dry and brown.
Throat: Coughing, throat blocked.
Stomach: Thirst and hunger, hiccoughs.
Male: Orchitis.
Respiratory: Dry cough, cannot breathe, wheezes, pants, voice gone, laryngitis.
Heart: Palpitation.
Skin: Itches, measles, pain.

Sleep: Terrors.
Fever: Heat and anxiety.

Squilla Maritima (Squilla or Scilla, Sea Onion).
Slow acting (several days), heart, kidney, lungs, mucous membranes, chronic bronchitis, dull rheumatic pains.
Eyes: Irritated.
Respiratory: Coughing, coryza, sneezing, may pass large quantities of urine when sneezing.
Urine: Involuntary spurting.
Skin: Prickly red spots all over body.
Better: Rest.
Worse: Motion.

Stannum Metallicum (Stan met, Tin).
Nervous and respiratory system, paralysis, weakness.
Head: Pains, ulcers.
Female: Prolapses.
Respiratory: Dry cough, puffing, chronic chest problems.
Extremities: Sudden collapse of limbs, dizziness and weakness, spasmodic twitching.

Staphysagria (Staph).
Anger, nervousness, irritability, frustration.
Mind: Peevish outbursts.
Eyes: Itchy, pain.
Throat: Difficulty swallowing.
Mouth: Black crumbling teeth, spongy bleeding gums.
Stomach: Canine hunger but flabby and weak.

Abdomen: Swollen with hot flatus, diarrhoea or constipation.

Female: Prolapses.

Skin: Eczema, scabs, dry itches, fig warts, nodes.

Extremities: Painful, stiff.

Stramonium (Stram, Thorn Apple, Datura Stramonium).

Brain, delirium, suppressed secretions and excretions, no pain, muscles immobile, graceful gentle motions, Parkinson's Disease.

Mind: Manic, delirious.

Head: Dizzy, staggers, falls.

Eyes: Wide staring, no vision.

Mouth: Dribbling, aversion to water, cannot swallow, jaw in constant motion.

Stomach: Vomits green bile, great thirst.

Urine: Suppression.

Sleep: Very disturbed.

Extremities: Rhythmic motion, staggering, twitching.

Streptococcinum (Strepto, Streptococci Bacteria).

Suppurative infections, sepsis, fevers, pharyngitis, tonsillitis, scarlet fever, impetigo, fasciitis, myositis (sore muscle), large number of virulent diseases. Frequently respiratory tract, bloodstream and skin, but skin may remain uninfected depending on the strain. Sinusitis, otitis (ear infection), and pneumonia may result. Cellulitis, joint or bone infections or meningitis or endocarditis (heart cavity), may result. Toxic shock syndrome may result from the system's reaction to streptococci in the system, or alternatively the bacteria may mimic molecules within the host, causing the host's immune system not to recognise it.

Strychninum (Strych, Alkaloid of Nux Vomica).

Motor centres and reflex actions of spinal cord, spasms, cramps, spasms of bladder, central nervous system, mental activities, sensors, respiration, stiff neck and face muscles, tetanic convulsions with relaxation between paroxysms, cannot be touched, stomach deranged, explosive sensations.

Head: Vertigo, jerking head up, itching.

Eyes: Protruding, staring, twitching, painful.

Ears: Burning, itching.

Face: Jaw closed in spasm.

Mouth: Violently itchy.

Stomach: Ceaseless retching and vomiting.

Abdomen: Terrible pains.

Rectum: Constipation, with explosive discharge.

Back: Stiff, spinal jerks.

Extremities: Convulsions, spasms, cramps.

Skin: Violent itch in nose, itching of whole body.

Sulphur (Sulph, Sublimated Sulphur).

Works from within to without, ending on skin, burning, itching worse for heat, worse for standing, dirty animals prone to skin infections, offensive discharges and breath, recurrent disease.

Mind: Delusions of own size, and irritability.

Head: Great itching and burning of skin.

Eyes: Burning ulceration of lids, burning eyes, ulceration of cornea.

Ears: Deafness.

Nose: Red, dry, scabs, dry catarrh, blocked, polyps.

Mouth: Tongue white, red on tip and sides, gums swollen, throbbing pains.

Throat: Seems blocked.

Stomach: Appetite non-existent or massive.

Abdomen: Painful to touch.

Rectum: Itching and burning, constipation, redness, oozing, prolapse.

Urine: Mucus and pus, burning.

Male: Stitches and itches.

Female: Itches and burns, nipples cracked.

Respiratory: Difficulty breathing, rattling.

Extremities: Trembling, pains, itching, burning bad smell, stiffness.

Sleep: Very disturbed.

Fever: Flashes, stinking.

Skin: Dry, scaly, suppurating, pimply pustules, itching, burning.

Symphytum (Symph, Comfrey, Knitbone).

Injuries to sinews, tendons and periosteum, joints, non – union of fractures, irritable stumps and bones at point of fracture, abscess and pain of periosteum.

Head: Inflammations of bone, red swellings.

Eye: For any traumatic injury of eye.

Tabacum (Tabac, Tobacco).

Throat, chest, bladder, rectum constricted. Breathless, deathly colour, diarrhoea, nausea, vomitting, ice-cold, giddy.

Head: Giddy.

Eyes: Blind, optic nerve atrophies.

Stomach: Really feeling sick.

Abdomen: Painfully distended.

Rectum: Paralysed, prolapse, diarrhoea, watery, stench, pain.

Urinary: Renal colic, pain.
Heart: Palpitation.
Respiratory: Dry cough, constricted.
Extremities: Ice cold, trembling, shuffling, feeble.
Fever: Chills.

Tarentula Hispania (Tarent, Spanish Spider).
Nerves, spine, restlessness, must keep moving, epilepsy.
Mind: Discontented, unpredictable.
Head: Vertigo.
Heart: Palpitations.
Female: Dry itch.
Extremities: Twitching, jerking, never still, trembling, yawning, contorting, weakness, numbness, multiple sclerosis.

Tellurium (Tell).
Slow developing, skin, ears, eyes, spine, odorous discharges, pains everywhere, skin, bones, tendons, joints.
Head: Itch, sensitive to touch.
Eyes: Red, cataracts, lesions, conjunctivitis, lids thick.
Ears: Itches, smells, discharges, deaf, infected behind.
Nose: Blocked, running, discharge down throat.
Rectum: Itch.
Body: Soreness and pains.
Skin: Odours, lesions, blotches, itches, stinging, eczema, ringworm.

Teucrium Marum (Teuc, Cat-thyme).
Nose and rectum, chronic catarrh, polyps, offensive crusts in nose.

Eyes: Swollen, red.

Ears: Discomfort.

Nose: Catarrh, polyps, discharge of large chunks, odour, foul breath, crawling feelings in nose with blockage.

Stomach: Vomitting green, huge appetite, permanent hiccough.

Respiratory: Dry cough, expectoration, bad taste.

Extremities: Tearing pains.

Rectum: Crawling sensation, ascarides, terrible itch.

Sleep: Disturbed, choking, starting.

Skin: Dry itch drives him crazy, cracked nails infected.

Theridion Currassavicum (Therid cur, Orange-back Spider).

Vertigo, aversion to noises, nausea, necrosis.

Mind: No interest or pleasure.

Head: Vertigo and vomitting.

Ears: Intolerant to noise.

Eyes: Averse to bright light.

Stomach: Nausea, vomitting, motion-sickness.

Back: Pain to touch.

Skin: Stinging, itching.

Worse: Touch, motion, noise.

Thuja Occidentalis (Thuja, Arbor Vitae).

Skin, blood, brain, kidneys, gastro-intestinal tract, characterised by growths of all sorts, some bleeding, some soft some hard, tumours to warts, to funguses, urinary organs and skin mainly affected, tearing pains, lameness, worse damp, moonlight problems, little energy, left sided, prevents suppuration so drives disease inwards.

Mind: Over-emotional.

Head: Scurf, greasy skin, stabbing pains.

Eyes: Iritis, eyes stuck at night from pus, eye tumours.

Ears: Discharge, polyps.

Nose: Green mucus with blood, ulcers, pain.

Mouth: Sore gums, tooth decay, blisters on tongue, pain.

Stomach: No appetite, eructations, flatulence, thirst.

Abdomen: Distended with indurations, gurgles, diarrhoea, forcible expulsion of flatus, constipation, haemorrhoids, anal fissures with warts, pain.

Urine: Pain, cannot empty bladder, dribbling, constant desire to urinate.

Female: Warts, pain, green discharge, polyps.

Respiratory: Hacking cough, worse for drinking water.

Extremities: Weakness, twitches, trembling, pain round paws and underneath, heels painful.

Skin: Tubercles, polyps, growths, ulcers, warts, bumps, blotches, herpes, pains, sensitive, cannot scratch.

Sleep: Unable to sleep.

Trillium Pendulum (Trill, White Beth-root).

Abortion threatens, bloody diarrhoea, faintness and dizziness, haemorrhages from inside, spitting blood, cramps.

Head: Nosebleed, confusion.

Stomach: Burning reflux.

Mouth: Gums loose and bleeding.

Rectum: Blood, diarrhoea.

Female: Prolapse and bleeding.

Respiratory: Coughing blood, sneezing, pain.

Tuberculinum (Tuber, Nosode from Tubercular Abscess). Only for use by qualified homeopath.

Skin, intestines, cystitis, tuberculosis, weak immunity, fatigue, emaciated, diarrhoea, trembling, arthritis, epilepsy, no motivation or endurance, ear, nose, throat infections.

Mind: Alternating mania and sadness, anger and depression, rages.

Head: Boils in nose, green pus, pains, poor sleep.

Ears: Offensive discharge.

Abdomen: Sudden diarrhoea, offensive, forcible ejection.

Respiratory: Suffocation, rattles, difficulty, bronchial problems, cough.

Skin: Terrible itch, psoriasis, measles.

Sleep: Cannot sleep at night, very tired all day.

Fever: Chilliness.

Better: Open air.

Typhoidinum (From morbid secretion).

Virulent bacteria carried in water and food and by carriers, intestine walls, blood, apparent influenza, fever, diarrhoea, blood discharge from rectum, delirium, collapse.

Mind: Confusion, delirium.

Tongue: Yellow-coated.

Pains: Head, throat, chest, abdomen, limbs, worse for any movement at all.

Exhaustion, chilled, restless, thirsty for small sips. Should be treated for symptoms, and a little salt and sugar added to water.

Urtica Urens (Urt u, Stinging Nettle).

All sorts of itches, needle jabs, crawling itch, discharge from mucous surfaces, spleen problems. Returns yearly at same time, uric acid. Rheumatism, skin eruptions.

Head: Vertigo, spleen problems.

Abdomen: Diseased intestine, massive secretions.

Male: Terrible itches.

Female: Bleeding, no milk.

Extremities: Pains.

Skin: Blotched, violent itches, nettle-rash, suppressed rash leading to rheumatism, burning, herpes.

Variolinum (Vario, Lymph from Small-pox Pustule).

Assists body immunity and recovery from pox virus.

Respiratory: Throat obstructed, difficult to breathe, aches everywhere.

Fever: Blazing hot, stinking.

Skin: Shingles, pustules, dry.

Veratrum album (Ver alb, White Hellebore).

Collapse, blueness, cold, weak pulse, purging, cramps, mania, mood switch.

Mind: Indifference alternating with howls and shrieks, pain.

Head: Neck cannot hold head up, vomitting, diarrhoea.

Eyes: Lustreless, no interest.

Face: No circulation, blue, collapsed look.

Tongue: Cold, pale, thirsty.

Stomach: Great hunger and thirst, vomitting straight up again.

Abdomen: Sensitive, cramps.

Rectum: Hot, constipation, forcible watery diarrhoea.

Respiratory: Weak, rattling, blocked, blue face, water causes cough.

Heart: Irregular, palpitations, weak, puffing.

Extremities: Neuralgic, swollen, sharp pains, cramps, cold, paralytic.

Skin: Ice cold, wrinkled, clammy.

Fever: Chill with thirst.

Worse: Night.

Better: Moving and warmth.

Vespa Crabo (Vesp, Live Wasp).

Skin and mucous membranes, dizziness when standing, fainting, nausea, bowel cramps.

Face: Conjunctivitis, swollen mouth and throat, burning pain.

Urine: Itching and burning.

Skin: Wheals, burning, itching, swellings, boils, relieved with white vinegar.

Yohimbinum (Yohimb, Coryanthe Yohimbe).

Central nervous system disease, stimulates lactation.

Head: Copious salivation, nausea.

Organs: Bleeding piles, intestinal haemorrhage, urethritis, erections.

Fever: Heat.

Sleep: Cannot sleep.

Zincum Metallicum (Zinc).

Neuralgia, pains in organs, hiccough, hysteria, epilepsy, heart pains.

Head: Intense pain.

Female: Pains from ovaries to feet.

Extremities: Spine and back pain intense, legs move incessantly, neuralgia in legs.

Zingiber (Ginger).

Kidneys cease function, digestion, respiratory and sexual close-down.

Nose: Terrible itch.

Stomach: Wind, rumbling, thirst.

Abdomen: Colic, diarrhoea, bloat, burning red anus.

Urine: Stinging, burning, stinking, suppressed, oozing.

Respiratory: Asthma, coughing, hawking.

Male: Very itchy.

Extremities: Weak, lame, cramps.

Glossary of Terms.

Abscess: Collection of pus caused by infection.

Acute: Arrives suddenly and energetically, departs as rapidly or becomes chronic.

Aggravation: Gets worse before it gets better.

Ameliorate: Makes less bad.

Allopathic: Orthodox medicines of opposites.

Atrophy: Wasting away.

Buboe: Enlarged, infected lymph node.

Canker: An open sore, not malignant, usually in mouth.

Caries: Holes in teeth, bone.

Catarrh: Inflamed nasal membrane resulting in runny nose and post-nasal drip.

Chancre: A highly infectious sore, being the first sign of a virulent disease.

Chi: Vital Force, Essence of Life.

Chronic: Slow developing, long lasting.

Constitutional remedy: The remedy which will cure all diseases in that constitution.

Dysentry: Severe diarrhoea with blood, as a result of a bacteria causing inflammation of the intestines.

Edema: Soft, puffy swellings under the skin.

Emphysema: Air sacs in lungs are enlarged and lose flexibility and breathing is impaired, with possible infection.

Epilepsy: Sudden losses or impairments of consciousness, sometimes with convulsions, due to irregular electrical pulses in the brain.

Eructations: Belching acid, with bits coming up.

Extremities: All legs or legs and arms.

Fig-wart: A little growth resembling a fig.

Flatus: Stomach gas.

Furuncle: Persistent, bacterially infected skin boil, spreading in numbers and affecting animals and fish, virulent and deadly.

Gangrene: Dead flesh from the blood supply being cut off.

Haemorrhage: Bleeding, running out.

Haemorrhoids: Painful, swollen veins in the rectum.

Hotspot: Itchy, burning, irritated spot of skin, often hairless.

Iatrogenisis: Disease caused by orthodox medicines.

Lesion: A wound resulting from illness or injury, sometimes infected.

Lymphangitis: Acute inflammation of lymph channels with red streaks under the skin.

Mania: A psychiatric disorder with excessive physical activity and obsessive compulsive behaviour.

Materia medica: All facts pertaining to a remedy.

Miasm: Nuclear memory of diseases from past generations, not genetic, curable with homeopathy.

Multiple sclerosis: An autoimmune disease affecting the brain and spinal cord.

Neuralgia: A very sore nerve, although the nerve does not change at all.

Opaque: Filmed over, cannot see through.

Orchitis: Bacterial or viral infection of testicles.

Palliative: Alleviating symptoms without affecting the cause.

Paralysis: Impairment of the ability to use voluntary muscles as usual.

Periosteum: Fibrous sheath covering bones, which has nerves and blood supply for the bones.

Symptom picture: All symptoms from emotional, mental, sidedness, modalities etc to the physical.

Photophobia: Aversion to, and fear of light.

Potentise: Dilute and succuss in homeopathic tradition, to increase power.

Psoriasis: Irritation and swelling of the skin, with itches, dryness and redness and silvery scales.

Reflect (remedies): The system cannot absorb more than it has at the present moment, and turns away any more.

Renal: Relating to the kidneys.

Repertorise: Collect all disease symptoms displayed by the patient, and match then as perfectly as possible to a remedy picture.

Scrofulous: Corrupt, degenerate, shabby, dirty.

Septicemia: Deadly infection of the blood, rapidly spreading to all parts of the body, life-threatening.

Simillimum: A medicine (remedy) which causes the same symptoms in a healthy patient as exist in the diseased patient one wishes to heal.

Sphincter: A circular muscle round a hole in the body, which it can open and close by expanding or contracting.

Succuss: Shake violently for two minutes.

Suppurate: Produces pus as a result of injury or infection.

Tetanus: Acute infection entering via wound, causing contractions and spasms around jaw and neck.

Urticaria: Skin rash with small red swellings.

Vital Force: Essence of Life, Chi.

Bibliography.

www.abchomeopathy.com
www.alonnissos.org
www.ambertech.com
www.blakkatz.com
www.cancernet.co.uk
www.christinachambreau.com
www.dogmark.com
www.druidry.org
www.ecovet.co.za
www.emofree.com
www.elixiers.com
www.harvestfields.ca
www.healthy.net
www.helios.co.uk
www.herbs2000.com
www.holistc-home.com
www.homeoint.com
www.homeopath.moonfruit.com
www.homeopathyhome.com
www.hpathy.com
www.islandnet.com
www.internethealthlibrary.com
www.mhra.gov.uk
www.lyghtforce.com
www.mediresource.sympatico.com
www.medicalhealthcures.com
www.ontariohomeopath.com

www.observer.guardian.co.uk
www.quantec.ch
www.realtime.net
www.ritecare.com
www.shirleys-wellness-cafe.com
www.simillimum.com
www.spiritindia.com
www.wholehealthmd.com

Allport, R. Homeopathy for your Pets. Wigmore Publications Ltd, London. 2000.

Ball, P. The Essence of Tao. Arcturus Publishing, London. 2004.

Boericke, W. Homoeopathic Materia Medica. Homoeopathic Books Service, Kent. 1999.

Buber, M. I and Thou. Simon and Shuster, London. 1996.

Castro, M. The Complete Homeopathic Handbook. Pan Books Ltd, London. 1996.

Chapman, E. How to use the 12 Tissue Salts. Thorsons, UK. 1979.

Culpeper. Complete Herbal. Wordsworth Edition, UK. 1995.

ECH General Assembly – XVII Symposium of GIRI 12-14 Nov 2004, Scientific Report.

Guide to Natural Healing. Geddes and Grosset, Scotland. 2005.

Hyne Jones, T.W. Dictionary of the Bach Flower Remedies. Saffron Walden, UK. 1995.

Kaptchuk, K. Chinese Medicine. Rider, London. 1983.

Kent, J.T. Repertory of the Homeopathic Materia Medica. B. Jain Publishers Pty Ltd, New Delhi. 2004.

Lockie, A. The Family Guide to Homeopathy. Hamish Hamilton, London. 1998.

Men's Health. Geddes and Grosset, Scotland. 2001.

Meyer, E. Family Encyclopaedia of Homeopathic Medicine. Bodywell Publishing. ?

Pert, J.C. Homeopathy. Wigmore Publications Ltd, London. 2002.

Pacaud, D. Homeopathy Encyclopedia. Hachette, London. 2003.

Reader's Digest. Natural Medicine. Readers Digest Association of South Africa (Pty) Limited, Cape Town. 1994.

Recognising Symptoms. Geddes and Grosset, Scotland. 2001.

Schneck, S. and Norris, N. The Complete Home Medical Guide for Cats. Scarborough House, New York. 1993.

White, H. Materia Medica Pharmacy, Pharmacology and Therapeutics. J. and A. Churchill, London. 1903.

Williams, T. Complete Chinese Medicine. Element Books Ltd, Dorset. 1999.

Womens' Health. Geddes and Grosset, Scotland. 2001.

www.ingramcontent.com/pod-product-compliance
Lightning Source LLC
Chambersburg PA
CBHW060448290526
45791CB00001B/25